P9-DEU-989

Living the Low Carb Life

POCKET

Carb Counter

JONNY BOWDEN, M.A., C.N.S.

Sterling Publishing Co., Inc.
New York

Published by Sterling Publishing Co., Inc.
387 Park Avenue South, New York, NY 10016

Text ©2005 by Jonny Bowden
Charts ©2005 by Sterling Publishing Co., Inc.
Nutrient Data compiled by Rebecca Lewis and Amy Mitchell

Distributed in Canada by Sterling Publishing
c/o Canadian Manda Group, 165 Dufferin Street
Toronto, Ontario, Canada M6K 3H6
Distributed in Great Britain by Chrysalis Books
64 Brewery Road, London N79NT, England
Distributed in Australia by Capricorn Link (Australia) Pty. Ltd.
P.O. Box 704, Windsor, NSW 2756, Australia

ISBN 1-4027-2509-4

Printed in Florida by Rose Printing Company

10 9 8 7 6 5 4 3 2 1

Data contained in the *Living the Low Carb Life Pocket Carb Counter* are based on information
published by the United States Department of Agriculture, the producers of brand-name
foods, and chain restaurants. Glycemic loads were calculated using glycemic index values
provided by www.glycemicindex.com and *The New Glucose Revolution* (Marlowe & Company).
Used with permission of Sydney University's Glycemic Index Research Service (SURGiS). Be
aware that nutritional values may vary depending upon the recipe used, and that products'
values may differ depending upon the region. Also, while data are accurate as of the time of
compilation, manufacturers may alter and update their recipes, and may discontinue products
as well as offer new ones.

Contents

Introduction

▓ Why You Need This Book and How to Use It

Welcome to the *Living the Low Carb Life Pocket Carb Counter*. I'm very proud of this little book because it goes into greater depth than any other carb or calorie counter currently on the market, hopefully without overwhelming you. Here you'll find all the foods you commonly eat, including some popular brand names. And while nutritional values vary somewhat from brand to brand, you'll get a good idea of whether or not that food is a healthy choice for your controlled-carbohydrate lifestyle. I hope the discussions of net carbs, sugar alcohols, and glycemic load clear up some confusion about low-carb living, and I also hope this book serves as a helpful general guide to making wise food choices.

A carb and calorie counter should be clear, easy to use, and not too crowded with unnecessary information. At the same time, it should tell you the important facts you need to know. The charts include essential points for each food: total calories, net carbs, protein, total fat, and fiber. I've also included my personal recommendation for every food entry, and, when available, the glycemic load rating. The glycemic load tells you the true impact a food has on your blood sugar, and is explained in depth on page 11. Not all foods have a glycemic load listing because only a relatively small number of foods have actually been tested; those that have been tested are mostly carbohydrate-rich foods, as these have the most impact on blood sugar.

I included a *total* fat column because I do not believe saturated fat should be singled out as the "bad" fat. More important is whether a fat is damaged or not—see "A Really Short Course in Fats" on page 13 for more information. Also, throughout the charts, I've indicated with an asterisk the foods that contain sugar alcohols to give you a heads-up if you're trying to avoid them (see page 9 for more information).

Then finally, there's the rating system.

It's not easy rating foods.

You'd think it would be, but believe me, it's not. Do you decide just based on the carb count? Absolutely not. That means a junk food made with chemicals and artificial sweeteners would get recommended just because its net carb count is low. And that's exactly the message I don't want to send.

And how about calories? If you're using this guide, you're probably concerned with either losing weight or maintaining your weight loss. Can I give a "Choose" rating to a food that is low in carbs but has 400 calories per serving? Not if I want to sleep at night.

Then there's the category problem. Can you rate cakes and cookies by the same standards as vegetables? Obviously, in the best of all possible worlds, you'd consume a ton of vegetables and eat cake once or twice a year on special occasions. But this is reality. So it's much more practical to rate each food group in comparison with its peers. I'd rather you didn't eat sweets at all—but you're going to (and for that matter, so am I). Therefore, my ratings for desserts, snacks, and fast foods are more about damage control than about recommending them as a healthy part of a low-carb diet. Some are just less bad than others.

Finally, there's the all-important issue of context. Take oils as an example. Some—like peanut oil—have a high smoke point (good) and are therefore not likely to be damaged if you're heating them to high temperatures. But that same oil has a very high concentration of omega-6 fats (which aren't so good). Conversely, some of the best oils from an omega-3 point of view—flaxseed oil, for example—are never to be used for cooking. These subtleties are not captured in a simple rating.

In the introduction to each section I've outlined a few points to be aware of when making food choices. Full disclosure: in many cases I used my clinical judgement based on years of advising clients about food, weight, and health. If pressed, I might not have a strictly objective reason for why one food received a "Restrict" rating and another an "In Moderation," simply because in many cases it's really close. When it was hard to decide, I simply went with my gut instinct and asked the questions, "Would I recommend this food to my family? And would I eat it myself?"

Also, make sure you're aware of the portion size that was used to compute the rating, and the glycemic load when it's available. Sometimes a food that is recommended in the 1/4-cup size wouldn't retain that recommendation if you ate a full cup of it. And vice versa. Some foods got low ratings because a normal portion size is way too high for a low-carb lifestyle, but if you eat a more reasonable portion, it's likely that some of those foods can be incorporated into your diet.

And last, but definitely not least: weight loss is different for every single person—sometimes maddeningly so. The stage of your program may influence whether a food is a good choice or not. For example, in the very early stages of weight loss, the majority of cereals are just not a good idea, but many of them received acceptable ratings in this book because once you're on maintenance—or if your personal carb tolerance allows it during ongoing weight loss—they won't do much damage. Those that scored an "Avoid" rating would probably not work even on maintenance.

Remember that you are unique, and even my ratings are not perfect. They're suggestions, and are meant to be used as a guide. And, as my dear friend Lee Bessinger says, "to eat consciously, you have to live consciously." Don't follow anyone blindly—even if it's me!

Enjoy the journey!

▩ Size Matters: The Truth About Portions, Carbs, and Calories

Americans don't seem to like complexity and nuance. Maybe it's the pace of our society, the influence of the MTV fast cut, or the speed of our Pentiums that has reprogrammed our brains and shortened our attention spans. Who knows? All I know is this: when it comes to nutrition information, people want it short, fast, and easy to understand.

Ah, were it that simple.

This desire for quick, easy answers is especially prevalent in the low-carb world, which has been all too quick to adopt the notion that losing weight is simply a matter of counting carbs. As H.L. Mencken once said, "For every complex problem there is a simple solution. And it is almost always wrong."

As those who read *Living the Low Carb Life* know, from the beginning of the twentieth century the playbook for weight loss consisted of one strategy: reduce calories. Enter Robert Atkins, who made a generation of frustrated dieters sit up and take notice. He maintained that carbohydrate-laden foods trigger an accelerated release of insulin, which in turn encourages fat storage, while limiting fat burning. According to Atkins, monitoring your carb intake forces your body to rely more heavily on fat as fuel; furthermore, limiting carbs cuts your appetite. Think about it, which are you more likely to do, eat six bowls of cereal while watching reruns of *Seinfeld* or pig out on brussels sprouts and steak? Atkins told us not to count calories (at least at first) and instead focus on the source of those calories. Millions of dieters found that they could eat more food than their previous Spartan low-fat diets had allowed, and still lose weight.

Ah, weight-loss nirvana. So far, so good.

This notion was given more credence when scientific studies started backing it up. For example, one important study placed obese teenage boys on one of two diets: either a conventional low-fat, calorie-controlled diet or the Atkins induction phase, in which carbs are limited to 20 grams a day. The low-fat group ate about 1,100 calories daily, while the Atkins group was permitted 1,800. And the Atkins group lost more weight.

Clearly, weight loss is about more than just calories. But, the whole thing went south when people began assuming that because calories aren't the whole picture, calories don't count *at all*.

One of the best studies to demonstrate that both carbohydrates and calories count was conducted by Dr. Penelope Green of Harvard University. She tested three groups: group one was put on a 1,500-calorie-per-day low-fat regimen and group two was put on a low-carb program and allowed an additional 300 daily calories. Group two—the low-carb, higher-calorie dieters—lost a bit more weight than the low-fat dieters, demonstrating that dieting is not just about calories. Then there was group number three: this was another low-carb group, but this group's calories were restricted to the 1,500 limit designated for the low-fat dieters. The result? This group lost more weight than any of them.

The point is this: you can't ignore calories. Eat too many of them, and you will stall or prevent weight loss on any diet. It's that simple. I've seen clients eat two whole chickens for dinner and then wonder what went wrong, because, after all, it was a "low-carb dinner." Sure, your low-carb plan will allow a bit more wiggle room than the standard low-fat diet, but don't think you can disregard quantity altogether just because your carb count is low.

I'm sorry. Don't shoot the messenger. I wish it were different.

Truth be told, we've gone too far in the opposite direction. Because we were so delighted by the revelation that calorie counting wasn't the only answer, we adopted the misconception that calories don't matter at all. They do. To get the best out of your controlled-carbohydrate eating plan, you need to pay attention to both carbs *and* calories.

Adjust your calorie intake to the amount suited for your particular metabolism, limit your carbs so you don't send your hormones (particularly insulin) into an orgy of fat storage, increase your fiber, and you've got the perfect nutritional trifecta.

Size—at least when it comes to portion—really does matter.

▨ What Are These Net Carbs, Anyway? And What About Sugar Alcohols?

Let's go back and think about the reasoning behind the low-carb approach.

Cutting carbohydrates gets us off the blood sugar roller coaster and helps control the body's insulin levels. By preventing huge spikes in blood sugar and the unhealthy sustained levels of insulin that follow, we're reversing the constant command to the body to "store that fat." And, of course, in addition to weight loss, we're also getting all the health benefits of lower triglycerides in the bargain.

But not all carbs are created equal, and not all have the same impact on blood sugar (see "The Blood Sugar Factor" on page 11 for more on this). In fact, some substances listed under carbohydrates on the nutrition facts label have no impact on blood sugar at all. Fiber is one example. If you take a glucose (blood sugar) reading and then drink a glass of pure psyllium husks or unsweetened Metamucil, when you measure your blood sugar again, the reading won't budge at all. Fiber simply has no effect on blood sugar because it's basically indigestible. Although it's grouped with the carbs on the nutrition facts label, we low carbers don't need to worry about it.

Enter the concept of net carbs. The idea is a good one: let's just count the carbohydrates we have to worry about, those that impact blood sugar and insulin. Also called "effective" or "impact" carbs, net carbs are simply the *total number of carbohydrate grams on the label, minus the fiber*. So, if you have a serving of raspberries that contains 14 grams of carbohydrate, but 8 of them are fiber, the net carbs equal 6. These are the ones you count. These are the ones that affect your blood sugar.

Atkins Nutritionals has developed its own wording, "Net Atkins Count," and is replacing the term net carbs on its products with the new phrase. The company recently did clinical tests in which they measured the blood sugar response to each of their products on average consumers. The Net Atkins Count is a number that represents the impact of each product on the average person's blood sugar. Meanwhile, net carbs remains the term used widely throughout the industry.

The low-carb diet revolution helped food manufacturers realize the market potential of low-carb products. And the use of sugar alcohols—the current darling of the low-carb world—provides manufacturers the opportunity to produce great-tasting foods that won't compromise a dieter's good intentions. Sugar alcohols, like maltitol, sorbitol, xylitol, mannitol, and erythritol, are sugar-free sweeteners that are regular, naturally occurring substances in food. Many of them don't cause sudden increases in blood sugar, and are instead slowly and incompletely absorbed through the small intestine into the blood, requiring little or no insulin. Manufacturers use sugar alcohols and related compounds—such as glycerin (a vegetable sweetener) and the fibers polydextrose and inulin—to improve their products' taste and because, unlike standard sweeteners, they seem to have no impact on blood sugar and insulin.

Is it true? Not exactly. Although the vegetable sweetener glycerin and the fiber polydextrose have little to no effect, sugar alcohols are another story. Their impacts vary. Maltitol, one of the most widely used sugar alcohols, does have a substantial effect on blood sugar. Erythritol and mannitol have no effect, and several others have some effect. Not only that, but diabetics may be particularly susceptible to those effects. And nondiabetics often experience extreme hunger one hour after consuming maltitol (cravings, anyone?). Atkins Nutritionals is currently working on reformulating their Endulge bars to limit the maltitol content, which is a very responsible thing to do.

And remember—sugar alcohols are not calorie free. They have between 0.2 (erythritol) and 3 (maltitol) calories per gram.

Then there's the other potential problem, just a theory at this point, but one that I frequently wonder about. Does the sweet taste of these products feed our cravings for sweets? Does it make us overeat? Is it possible that, perhaps through a conditioned response, our insulin levels respond to the very taste of something sweet, even though there's no actual physiological stimulus for it to do so? Food for thought.

I think the concept of net carbs is a good one, but I'm hesitant to be too cavalier about subtracting all sugar alcohols from total carbs as part of the calculation. Remember, some people even have sugar reactions to sweeteners like Splenda and aspartame—so maybe we shouldn't completely ignore sugar alcohols until we know more. Glycerin, polydextrose, erythritol, and mannitol look like the safest bets right now, and if you're not diabetic you should be fine with xylitol. My suggestion: count half the grams of sugar alcohols as part of your total carb content. That will give you a few more grams than the net carb count on the label, but you'll be playing it safe.

▨ The Blood Sugar Factor: The Truth About the Glycemic Index and the Glycemic Load

In this book, we use the glycemic load rather than the glycemic index to indicate the foods that are conducive to weight loss. Here's why: the glycemic index is a useless number.

Now, you've probably heard different. You've heard that the glycemic index is a measure of how much and how quickly specific foods raise your blood sugar (true). And you've probably heard that it's also a good way to determine which foods will suit your low-carb diet (*not* true). While it's absolutely essential to know how a food will impact your blood sugar and your insulin level, the glycemic index, unfortunately, doesn't tell you that.

The glycemic *load*, however, does.

The glycemic index of a food is like the price tag on a pound of spices. Let's say you go into an exotic spice store and spot an unusual spice selling for 300 dollars a pound. "Three hundred bucks a pound!" you say. "That's expensive!" Well, that's true. But knowing the price per pound won't tell you how much your bill at the cash register is going to be—and that's what you really want to know. Let's say you go and purchase ¼ teaspoon of the exotic spice, which is all you need for the dish you're preparing. You hit the checkout counter and the bill is only...fifty-five cents!

Similarly, the glycemic index alone won't tell you the "cost" to your blood sugar. If you want to know the impact a food will have on your blood sugar and insulin level, you have to know more than just its glycemic index: you have to know the portion size. The glycemic load takes both index *and* portion size into account and gives you a much more meaningful number. Let me explain.

The glycemic index is a measure of how much a fifty-gram portion of a carbohydrate food will raise your blood sugar, compared with a fixed amount of pure sugar (glucose) or white bread. Carrots, which have a high glycemic index, are a perfect example of why the index alone is a useless number.

Remember our example about the price of spices? The glycemic index is a measure of the price, but the glycemic load—a far more important measure—tells you what you're actually going to pay when it comes time to tally up. The glycemic load takes into account how much you're actually "buying," not just the price per pound. Carrots, for example, which have a glycemic index of ninety-two, seem "expensive"—but remember, that's for a fifty-gram serving! There are only three or four net carbs in one carrot. To get any serious blood sugar spike you'd have to eat about a dozen whole carrots. As the wonderful nutritionist and botanist at the USDA, Dr. C. Leigh Broadhurst, once said, "Nobody ever became diabetic on peas and carrots."

Now, a food may have both a high glycemic index *and* a high glycemic load. That would be a food to avoid. And some foods with a low glycemic rating actually raise insulin levels more than you'd guess from the numbers (eggs and milk are examples, though we're not 100 percent sure why). But, by and large, the glycemic load ratings provided in the following charts can help guide you in choosing the right foods to maintain healthy blood sugar levels. For maximum weight loss, and to minimize the impact on your blood sugar, choose foods that have a "Low" glycemic load rating.

And remember: because the glycemic load takes portion size into account, the glycemic load ratings (low, medium, or high) only apply to the serving sizes listed. If you eat a larger portion, the load will be higher.

▩ A Really Short Course in Fats

Here's the deal with fats—I'm going to explain it with an absolute minimum of biochemistry, I promise. Think of fats like bricks. Bricks come in different colors—red, gray, and white, plus some variations. Fats also come in different "colors," except they're classified according to their chemical structure (i.e., their saturation). There's another similarity between fats and bricks: both are used for building things. The body uses fatty acids to construct and strengthen structures such as cell membranes, hormones, and even the brain.

Fats are categorized based upon their stiffness: saturated fats tend to be stiffer (they're solid at room temperature), while unsaturated fats are more fluid (like fish oil or nut oil). The truth is, if you're building something as important as the human body, you need both. Membranes, for example, have to be stiff enough to protect the contents of the cell, yet fluid enough to allow for communication and movement between cells.

In addition to building membranes, fats are also used to build hormones called eicosanoids. Eicosanoids come in several "flavors," which need to be balanced for optimum health. For example, some eicosanoids are pro-inflammatory and some are anti-inflammatory. This is where the right fats come in. The pro-inflammatory eicosanoid hormones are produced by omega-6 fats, while anti-inflammatory hormones are a product of omega-3s. We get plenty of omega-6s from our diet, but nowhere near enough of the crucial omega-3s. In fact, many nutritionists believe that this lack of balance is one of the major problems in the American diet and is responsible for a host of health woes.

Omega-3 fats have been shown to have anti-cancer properties. They've been used in the treatment of bipolar depression. They absolutely lower triglycerides, which, as you know from *Living the Low Carb Life*, increase the risk of heart disease. Omega-3s are protective of the heart, good for circulation, and they lower blood pressure. The amount of research on omega-3 fats is so massive at this point that virtually everyone in the health sciences—even the most nutritionally unaware—has heard about them. And practically everyone recommends them.

Another interesting thing about omega-3 fats: two of them, DHA (docosahexanoic acid) and EPA (eicosapentaenoic acid), are made inside the body from the third, ALA (alpha-linolenic acid). You can't make your own alpha-linolenic acid—you must get it from food or supplements, which is why it's known as an "essential fat." ALA is the main reason people take flaxseed oil, though the flax itself is even better because it also contains fiber and other nutrients. But here's the thing: only about 20 percent of the ALA you eat gets converted to the other two omega-3s, the very important DHA and EPA. That's why I always recommend taking the ready-made stuff—DHA and EPA, either from fish-oil supplements or from fish directly. Of course, recent discoveries about pollution in farmed fish make it even more imperative that you get your fish and fish oil from tested, pristine sources.

In addition to omega-3s, there are other important fats to be aware of. The very heart-healthy omega-9s are found in oils like extra virgin olive oil and macadamia nut oil. Certain saturated fatty acids—especially those found in coconut oil—are extremely beneficial for the human body. So are reasonable amounts of saturated fat from whole natural foods like butter and eggs. It's almost never necessary to supplement with omega-6s because we get more than enough of them in our diet (with the possible exception of the omega-6 known as GLA (gamma-linolenic acid), which is found in evening primrose oil and borage oil). Omega-6 is the principal fat in processed purified cooking oils like safflower, sunflower, and corn oil, which I recommend you throw out of your kitchen cabinet.

Ideally, we should get a nice blend of fats: some saturated for their stiffness, their boost to HDL cholesterol, and their benefits on other fronts; lots of omega-3s; a healthy dollop of omega-9s; and a modest intake of omega-6s, preferably from cold-pressed organic oils.

The one fat we should avoid at all costs? Trans-fats. Except for the absolutely tiny amount naturally found in the fat of some ruminants, trans-fats are the worst thing on the planet. A committee of scientific experts studied trans-fats at the request of the USDA and concluded that the acceptable human intake of trans-fats was zero. Enough said?

The take-home point: fats, like bricks, are essential tools used to build a strong, healthy body. And the better the bricks, the better the building.

Beverages

I DON'T NEED TO TELL YOU THAT THE BEST DRINK ON THE PLANET IS water. But I will anyway. When cells dehydrate, sodium and potassium levels are affected, which can mess with metabolic processes. A large number of the symptoms we deal with on a daily basis—including fatigue, migraines, heartburn, and arthritis—could be relieved by simply drinking more water. No kidding.

What if you don't like water? Get over it. There's just no substitute—would you wash your clothes in soda? But there's good news: a new company called Flavors To Go (www.Flavors2Go.com) has a terrific line of calorie-free flavored syrups. You can add a few drops to your water for a change in taste without adding any carbs or calories.

Now let's talk about the other stuff. Some of it's easy. Soda: bad. Period. Fruit juice, same thing: pure sugar, with little redeeming nutritional value. Coffee is acceptable, but you shouldn't overdo it. The absolute perfect drink is green tea, which not only has the potential to help with weight loss, but contains a cornucopia of cancer-fighting phytonutrients your body will love. Drink it often.

And then there's alcohol. Wine (particularly red wine) has a lot of benefits, due mainly to a compound called resveratrol, thought to fight the plaque that can block arteries. But wine also has a dark side: the calories add up quickly and fat burning stalls when alcohol is being processed in the body. Enjoy it, but don't overindulge. Dr. Richard Bernstein, author of *The Diabetes Solution,* allows his clients one beer a day, but no more. Spirits—gin, rum, vodka, and whiskey—have no carbs, but have all the problems associated with alcohol. Enjoy them, but get familiar with the term "moderation." And cross those liqueurs and mixed drinks off your list altogether.

BEVERAGES

Food	Cal	Net Carb	Protein	Fiber	Total Fat	Glycemic Load	Advice
Alcoholic Beverages							
beer, light, 12 oz	99	4.6	0.7	0	0	ND	🍴
beer, regular, 12 oz	146	12.8	1.1	0.4	0	ND	⊘
liquors, 1 oz serving							
coffee liqueur, 53 proof	117	16.3	0	0	0.1	ND	⊘
coffee liqueur, 63 proof	107	11.2	0	0	0.1	ND	⊘
crème de menthe, 72 proof	125	14	0	0	0.1	Low	⊘
gin, rum, vodka, whiskey, 80 proof	64	0	0	0	0	Low	🍴
mixed/frozen drinks							
daiquiri, 8 oz	448	16.4	0	0.4	0	ND	⊘
martini, 4 oz	276	2.4	0	0	0	ND	⊘
piña colada, 8 oz	437	56.1	1.1	0.8	4.7	ND	⊘
wine, 4 oz serving							
dessert, dry	179	13.8	0.2	0	0	Low	⊘
dessert, sweet	189	16.2	0.2	0	0	Low	⊘
light	59	1.4	0.6	0	0	Low	🍴
nonalcoholic	7	1.3	0.6	0	0	Low	🍴🍴
red	85	2	0.2	0	0	Low	🍴

ND = No Data

Food	Cal	Net Carb	Protein	Fiber	Total Fat	Glycemic Load	Advice
rosé	84	1.7	0.2	0	0	Low	⚕
sake (rice wine)	156	5.8	0.6	0	0	ND	⊘
white	80	0.9	0.1	0	0	Low	⚕
Carbonated Beverages, 12 oz serving							
club soda	0	0	0	0	0	ND	⚕⚕⚕
cola	155	39.8	0.2	0	0	High	⊘
cola, low-calorie w/aspartame	4	0.4	0.4	0	0	ND	⚕
cola, low-calorie w/sodium saccharin	0	0.4	0	0	0	ND	⚕
ginger ale	124	32.1	0	0	0	ND	⊘
lemon-lime soda	147	38.3	0	0	0	High	⊘
orange	179	45.8	0	0	0	High	⊘
root beer	152	39.2	0	0	0	ND	⊘
tonic water	124	32.2	0	0	0	ND	⊘
carbonated beverages, restaurant-size							
Coca-Cola Classic, 1 medium (21 fl oz)	210	58	0	0	0	High	⊘
Diet Coke, any size	0	0	0	0	0	ND	⚕
Sprite, 1 medium (21 fl oz)	210	56	0	0	0	High	⊘

 Avoid   Restrict   In Moderation   Choose

Food	Cal	Net Carb	Protein	Fiber	Total Fat	Glycemic Load	Advice
Chocolate-flavored Beverages							
beverage mix, powder, prepared w/whole milk, 8 oz	226	30.6	8.6	1.1	8.6	ND	🍴⃠
chocolate milk, chocolate syrup w/whole milk, 8 oz	254	35.2	8.7	0.8	8.4	ND	🍴
cocoa mix, powder, 1 packet prepared w/water, 6 oz	113	23	1.7	1	1.1	Med.	🍴⃠
cocoa mix, w/aspartame, powder, prepared w/water, 6 oz	56	9.4	2.4	1	0.4	ND	🍴
Nestlè Carnation hot cocoa mix w/marshmallows, 1 packet	112	23.8	1.4	0.5	1	Med.	🍴⃠
Nestlè Carnation hot cocoa mix, no sugar added, 1 packet	55	7.6	4.3	0.8	0.4	ND	🍴
Swiss Miss Cocoa mix, low-calorie, w/aspartame, powder, 1 packet	54	8.5	3.8	0.2	0.5	ND	🍴
Coffee Beverages							
brewed							
espresso, regular or decaf, restaurant-prepared, 1 fl oz	1	0	0	0	0	ND	🍴🍴
from grounds, regular or decaf, 8 oz	9	0	0.3	0	0	ND	🍴🍴
instant							
decaffeinated, powder, prepared w/water, 8 oz	5	1	0.3	0	0	ND	🍴🍴
regular, prepared w/water, 8 oz	5	0.8	0.2	0	0	ND	🍴🍴
substitute, cereal grain beverage, prepared w/water, 8 oz	12	1.7	0.2	0.7	0.1	ND	🍴🍴
Dairy-based Beverages							
eggnog, 1 cup	343	34.4	9.7	0	19	ND	🍴⃠

Food	Cal	Net Carb	Protein	Fiber	Total Fat	Glycemic Load	Advice
eggnog-flavored mix, powder, prepared w/whole milk, 8 oz	258	38.6	8	0	8.2	ND	
shake, fast food, chocolate, 10 oz	264	38.6	7.1	4	7.7	ND	
shake, fast food, strawberry, 10 oz	320	52.4	9.6	1.1	7.9	ND	
shake, fast food, vanilla, 10 oz	231	37	7.3	0.2	6.2	ND	
Flavored Water, 8 fl oz							
Fruit2O	0	0	0	0	0	ND	
Vitamin Water	50	13	0	0	0	ND	
Fruit-flavored Beverages							
fruit-flavored drinks, canned, 8 oz serving							
fruit punch drink, w/added nutrients	117	29.2	0	0.5	0	Med.	
grape drink	112	28.9	0	0	0	ND	
orange drink	126	32	0	0	0	ND	
fruit-flavored, frozen concentrate, prepared w/water, 8 oz serving							
fruit punch drink	114	28.6	0.2	0.2	0	Med.	
lemonade	131	33.9	0.2	0.2	0.2	ND	
orange drink, breakfast type, w/juice and pulp	112	28.3	0.3	0	0	Med.	
fruit-flavored, powder, prepared w/water							
fruit punch-flavored drink, 8 oz	97	24.8	0	0	0	ND	
lemonade, 8 oz	103	26.9	0	0	0	ND	

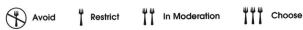

Avoid   Restrict   In Moderation   Choose

Food	Cal	Net Carb	Protein	Fiber	Total Fat	Glycemic Load	Advice
lemonade mix, Kraft Country Time w/vitamin C, 1 serving	64	17.7	0	0	0.2	ND	⊘
lemonade, low-calorie, w/aspartame, 8 oz	5	1.2	0.1	0	0	ND	⟊
orange-flavored drink, low-calorie, breakfast type, 8 oz	5	2.1	0	0.1	0	ND	⟊
orange-flavored drink, breakfast type, 8 oz	133	34	0	0.3	0	ND	⟊
sugar-free Kraft Country Time pink lemonade mix, w/vitamin C, 1 serving	5	1.7	0.1	0	0	ND	⟊
sugar-free, low-calorie Kraft, Crystal Light soft drink mix, lemonade, 1 serving	5	0.2	0.1	0	0	ND	⟊
bottled, ready-to-drink							
Powerade Mountain Blast, 1 child (12 fl oz)	70	18	0	0	0	High	⊘
Powerade Mountain Blast, 1 small (16 fl oz)	100	25	0	0	0	High	⊘
Powerade Mountain Blast, 1 medium (21 fl oz)	140	36	0	0	0	High	⊘
Powerade Mountain Blast, 1 large (32 fl oz)	200	53	0	0	0	High	⊘
Snapple, Kiwi Strawberry Cocktail, 8 oz	117	28.8	0.2	0	0	ND	⊘
thirst quencher drink, 8 oz	60	15.2	0	0	0	Med.	⊘
thirst quencher drink, low-calorie, 8 oz	26	7.2	0	0	0	ND	⊘
Juices, 8 oz							
apple juice, canned or bottled, unsweetened	117	28.8	0.2	0.2	0.3	Med.	⊘
carrot juice, 1 cup	94	20	2.2	1.9	0.4	43	⟊
cranberry juice, unsweetened	116	30.5	1	0.3	0.3	ND	⊘

Food	Cal	Net Carb	Protein	Fiber	Total Fat	Glycemic Load	Advice
grape juice, canned or bottled, unsweetened, w/o added vitamin C	154	37.5	1.4	0.3	0.2	ND	⊗
grapefruit juice, canned, unsweetened	94	22	1.3	0.2	0.3	Med.	⊺
orange juice, canned, unsweetened	104	24	1.5	0.5	0.4	Med.	⊗
pineapple juice, canned, unsweetened	140	34	0.8	0.5	0.2	Med.	⊗
prune juice, canned	182	42.1	1.6	2.6	0.1	ND	⊗
tomato juice, canned, w/salt added	41	9.3	1.8	1	0.1	Low	⊺
tomato juice, canned, w/o added salt	41	9.3	1.9	1	0.1	Low	⊺
vegetable juice cocktail, canned	46	9.1	1.5	1.9	0.2	ND	⊺
Juice Drinks, 8 oz serving unless noted							
cranberry juice cocktail, bottled	144	36.1	0	0.3	0.3	ND	⊗
cranberry juice cocktail, low-calorie, bottled, w/calcium, saccharin, and corn sweetener	45	10.9	0.1	0	0	ND	⊗
cranberry-apple juice drink, bottled	174	44.2	0.2	0.2	0.1	ND	⊗
cranberry-apple juice drink, low-calorie, w/vitamin C added	46	11.1	0.2	0.2	0	ND	⊗
fruit punch juice drink, frozen concentrate, prepared w/water	124	30.1	0.3	0.2	0.5	ND	⊗
grape juice drink, canned	125	32	0.3	0	0	ND	⊗
orange juice drink	132	33.3	0.5	0	0	ND	⊗

 Avoid   ⊺ Restrict   ⊺⊺ In Moderation   ⊺⊺⊺ Choose

Food	Cal	Net Carb	Protein	Fiber	Total Fat	Glycemic Load	Advice
Tea							
black tea, regular and decaf, 6 oz	2	0.5	0	0	0	ND	⊡
green tea, 6 oz	0	0	0	0	0	ND	⊡⊡⊡
herb, chamomile, brewed, 6 oz	2	0.4	0	0	0	ND	⊡⊡⊡
herb, other than chamomile, brewed, 6 oz	2	0.4	0	0	0	ND	⊡⊡⊡
iced tea							
instant, sweetened, lemon-flavored, w/o added ascorbic acid, powder, 8 oz	88	22.1	0.1	0	0.1	ND	⊘
instant, unsweetened, lemon-flavored, prepared, 8 oz	5	1.0	0	0	0	ND	⊡
lemon-flavored, Nestlè, Nestea ready-to-drink, 8 oz	89	20.4	0	0	0	ND	⊘
sugar-free, Kraft Crystal Light, low-calorie mix, w/aspartame, powdered, 1 serving	3	0.4	0.1	0	0	ND	⊡

Dairy and Eggs

THIS CATEGORY CONTAINS A VARIETY OF FOODS, SOME OF THEM absolutely terrific and others that can be problematic.

Let's start with the good news: eggs. In my opinion, eggs just might be one of nature's most perfect foods, and I'm a big fan of the whole egg, including the nutritious yolk. I strongly recommend eggs from free-range chickens that are also hormone-free. It's pretty easy to find them these days, and they're worth the extra money. Be aware that eggs are a common source of food sensitivities. And believe it or not, eggs can raise insulin levels—though nowhere near as much as carbohydrate-laden foods.

I'm not such a fan of milk, which is also very allergenic for some people. In my opinion, it's just not a necessary food in the human diet. Milk also has a tendency to raise insulin, even though the carb content is modest. You can definitely get your calcium elsewhere—from sardines or green/leafy vegetables, for example. Even Swiss cheese is a viable source! But if you are going to drink milk, you should go organic.

Cheese is a perfectly good food but is also one of the chief culprits in stalling weight loss for many dieters. It's very high in calories and very easy to overeat. Be aware, and consume it consciously.

I have no problem with small amounts of cream or half and half, but I'd recommend you avoid the powdered "creamers" at all costs because they're loaded with trans-fats. Just as with butter, you're way better off choosing the real thing than a highly processed substitute.

DAIRY AND EGGS

Food	Cal	Net Carb	Protein	Fiber	Total Fat	Glycemic Load	Advice
Cheese, 1 oz unless noted							
blue cheese	100	0.7	6.1	0	8.2	Low	♈♈♈
brick	105	0.8	6.6	0	8.4	Low	♈♈♈
Brie	95	0.1	5.9	0	7.9	Low	♈♈♈
Camembert	85	0.1	5.6	0	6.9	Low	♈♈♈
caraway	107	0.9	7.1	0	8.3	Low	♈♈♈
cheddar	114	0.4	7.1	0	9.4	Low	♈♈♈
cheddar or Colby, low-fat	49	0.5	6.9	0	2	Low	♈♈♈
Cheshire	110	1.4	6.6	0	8.7	Low	♈♈♈
Colby	112	0.7	6.7	0	9.1	Low	♈♈♈
cottage cheese, 1/2 cup							
creamed	108	2.8	13.1	0	4.7	Low	♈♈♈
creamed, w/ fruit	110	5	12.1	0.2	4.4	Low	♈♈♈
low-fat, 1% milkfat	81	3.1	14	0	1.2	Low	♈♈♈
low-fat, 2% milkfat	102	4.1	15.5	0	2.2	Low	♈♈♈
nonfat, uncreamed, dry	96	2.1	19.5	0	0.5	Low	♈♈♈
cream cheese, 1 tbsp	51	0.4	1.1	0	5.1	Low	♈♈♈
cream cheese, fat-free, 1 tbsp	14	0.8	2.1	0	0.2	Low	♈♈♈

ND = No Data

Food	Cal	Net Carb	Protein	Fiber	Total Fat	Glycemic Load	Advice
cream cheese, low-fat, 1 tbsp	35	1.1	1.6	0	2.6	Low	♈♈♈
Edam	101	0.4	7.1	0	7.9	Low	♈♈♈
feta	75	1.2	4	0	6	Low	♈♈♈
fontina	110	0.4	7.3	0	8.8	Low	♈♈♈
goat cheese, hard	128	0.6	8.7	0	10.1	Low	♈♈
goat cheese, semisoft	103	0.7	6.1	0	8.5	Low	♈♈♈
goat cheese, soft	76	0.3	5.3	0	6	Low	♈♈♈
Gouda	101	0.6	7.1	0	7.8	Low	♈♈♈
gruyère	117	0.1	8.5	0	9.2	Low	♈♈
Limburger	93	0.1	5.7	0	7.7	Low	♈♈♈
Mexican, queso anejo	106	1.3	6.1	0	8.5	Low	♈♈♈
Mexican, queso asadero	101	0.8	6.4	0	8	Low	♈♈♈
Mexican, queso chihuahua	106	1.6	6.1	0	8.4	Low	♈♈♈
Monterey	106	0.2	6.9	0	8.6	Low	♈♈♈
Monterey, low-fat	88	0.2	7.9	0	6.1	Low	♈♈♈
mozzarella							
nonfat	42	0.5	8.9	0.5	0	Low	♈♈♈
part skim milk	82	0.8	6.9	0	4.5	Low	♈♈♈

 Avoid   Restrict   In Moderation   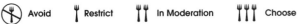 Choose

Food	Cal	Net Carb	Protein	Fiber	Total Fat	Glycemic Load	Advice
whole milk	85	0.6	6.3	0	6.3	Low	♟♟♟
Muenster	104	0.3	6.6	0	8.5	Low	♟♟♟
Muenster, low-fat	77	1	6.9	0	4.9	Low	♟♟♟
Neufchatel	74	0.8	2.8	0	6.6	Low	♟♟♟
Parmesan, grated, 1 tbsp	22	0.2	1.9	0	1.4	Low	♟♟♟
Parmesan, hard	111	0.9	10.1	0	7.3	Low	♟♟♟
port du salut	100	0.2	6.7	0	8	Low	♟♟♟
processed cheese							
American, low-fat, pasteurized	50	1	6.9	0	2	Low	♟♟♟
American cheddar, imitation	67	3.3	4.7	0	3.9	Low	🚫
cheddar or American, pasteurized, fat-free	41	3.8	6.3	0	0.2	Low	♟♟♟
pimento, pasteurized	106	0.5	6.3	0	8.9	Low	♟♟♟
Swiss, low-fat, pasteurized	48	1.2	7.1	0	1.4	Low	♟♟♟
provolone	100	0.6	7.3	0	7.6	Low	♟♟♟
ricotta, part skim milk	39	1.5	3.2	0	2.2	Low	♟♟♟
ricotta, whole milk	49	0.9	3.2	0	3.6	Low	♟♟♟
Romano	110	1	9	0	7.6	Low	♟♟
Roquefort	105	0.6	6.1	0	8.7	Low	♟♟

Food	Cal	Net Carb	Protein	Fiber	Total Fat	Glycemic Load	Advice
soy cheeses (see also Legumes)							
soy cheese, 1 oz	60	6	3	0	2	ND	ᵜᵜᵜ
sandwich slices, Soya Kaas, 1 slice	40	0	4	0	3	ND	ᵜᵜᵜ
sandwich slices, Soyco, 1 slice	60	1	6	0	3	ND	ᵜᵜᵜ
cream cheese, Soya Kaas Natural Cream Cheese Alternative, plain, 2 tbsp	80	0	3	0	9	ND	ᵜᵜᵜ
cream cheese, Tofutti Better than Cream Cheese, plain, 2 tbsp	120	13	1	0	7	ND	ᵜ
Swiss	108	1.5	7.6	0	7.9	Low	ᵜᵜ
Swiss, low-fat	50	1	8	0	1.4	Low	ᵜᵜᵜ
Tilsit	96	0.5	6.9	0	7.4	Low	ᵜᵜᵜ
Cream, 1 tbsp unless noted							
dessert topping, powdered, 1 oz	162	14.7	1.4	0	11.2	ND	
dessert topping, pressurized	11	0.6	0	0	0.9	ND	ᵜᵜ
half and half	20	0.7	0.4	0	1.7	ND	ᵜᵜᵜ
half and half, fat-free	9	1.4	0.4	0	0.2	ND	ᵜᵜᵜ
heavy whipping	52	0.4	0.3	0	5.6	ND	ᵜᵜᵜ
light (coffee cream or table cream)	29	0.6	0.4	0	2.9	ND	ᵜᵜᵜ
light whipping	44	0.4	0.3	0	4.6	ND	ᵜᵜᵜ
whipped cream topping, pressurized	8	0.4	0.1	0	0.7	ND	ᵜᵜᵜ

 Avoid   ᵜ Restrict   ᵜᵜ In Moderation   ᵜᵜᵜ Choose

Food	Cal	Net Carb	Protein	Fiber	Total Fat	Glycemic Load	Advice
cream substitute							
liquid, 1 fl oz	41	3.4	0.3	0	3	ND	🚫
liquid, light, 1 fl oz	21	2.7	0.2	0	1.1	ND	🚫
powdered, 1 tsp	11	1.1	0.1	0	0.7	ND	🚫
powdered, light, 1 tsp	9	1.5	0	0	0.3	ND	🚫
soy creamer, Silk, plain, 1 tbsp	15	1	0	0	1	ND	🍴🍴🍴
sour cream							
cultured	26	0.5	0.4	0	2.5	ND	🍴🍴🍴
reduced-fat	27	1.1	1.1	0	2.1	ND	🍴🍴🍴
reduced-fat, cultured	20	0.6	0.4	0	1.8	ND	🍴🍴🍴
light	20	1.1	0.5	0	1.6	ND	🍴🍴🍴
fat-free	11	2.3	0.5	0	0	ND	🍴🍴🍴
imitation	31	1	0.4	0	2.9	ND	🚫

Eggs and Egg Dishes

Food	Cal	Net Carb	Protein	Fiber	Total Fat	Glycemic Load	Advice
eggs							
1 extra large	85	0.5	7.3	0	5.8	Low	🍴🍴🍴
1 jumbo	96	0.5	8.2	0	6.5	Low	🍴🍴🍴
1 large	74	0.4	6.3	0	5	Low	🍴🍴🍴
1 medium	65	0.3	5.5	0	4.4	Low	🍴🍴🍴
1 small	54	0.3	4.7	0	3.7	Low	🍴🍴🍴

Food	Cal	Net Carb	Protein	Fiber	Total Fat	Glycemic Load	Advice
egg white, 1 large	17	0.2	3.6	0	0.1	Low	YYY
egg yolk, 1 large	55	0.6	2.7	0	4.5	Low	YYY
duck, 1 egg	130	1	9	0	9.6	Low	YY
goose, 1 egg	266	1.9	20	0	19.1	Low	Y
quail, 1 egg	14	0	1.2	0	1	Low	YYY
turkey, 1 egg	135	0.9	10.8	0	9.4	Low	YY
egg dishes							
eggnog, 1 cup	343	34.4	9.7	0	19	ND	⊗
fried egg, 1 large egg	92	0.4	6.3	0	7	ND	YYY
hard-boiled egg, 1 large egg	78	0.6	6.3	0	5.3	ND	YYY
omelet, 1 large egg	93	0.4	6.5	0	7.3	ND	YYY
scrambled egg, 1 large egg	101	1.3	6.8	0	7.5	ND	YYY
egg substitutes							
frozen, 1/4 cup	96	1.9	6.8	0	6.7	ND	⊗
liquid, 1/4 cup	53	0.4	7.5	0	2.1	ND	⊗
powder, 1 oz	129	6.3	16.1	0	3.8	ND	⊗
Milk							
buttermilk, dried, 1 tbsp	25	3.2	2.2	0	0.4	ND	YYY

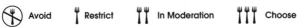

⊗ Avoid   Y Restrict   YY In Moderation   YYY Choose

Food	Cal	Net Carb	Protein	Fiber	Total Fat	Glycemic Load	Advice
buttermilk, low-fat, 1 cup	98	11.7	8.1	0	2.2	ND	ψ
buttermilk, reduced-fat, 1 cup	137	13	10	0	4.9	ND	ψ
canned, condensed, sweetened, 1 fl oz	123	20.8	3	0	3.3	Med.	⊘
canned, evaporated, nonfat, 1 fl oz	25	3.6	2.4	0	0.1	ND	ψψψ
canned, evaporated, 1 fl oz	42	3.2	2.2	0	2.4	ND	ψψψ
chocolate milk, 1 cup	208	23.9	7.9	2	8.5	Med.	⊘
chocolate milk, low-fat, 1 cup	158	24.9	8.1	1.2	2.5	Low	⊘
dry, nonfat, instant, 1/3 cup (makes 1 cup)	82	12	8.1	0	0.2	ND	ψψ
dry, nonfat, regular, 1/4 cup	109	15.6	10.9	0	0.2	ND	ψ
dry, whole, 1/4 cup	159	12.3	8.4	0	8.6	ND	ψ
goat milk, 1/2 cup	84	5.5	4.4	0	5.1	ND	ψψψ
low-fat, 1% milkfat, 1 cup	102	12.2	8.2	0	2.4	ND	ψψ
milk substitutes							
chai, soymilk, Silk, 1 cup	140	19	6	0	4	Low	ψ
chocolate, soymilk, Silk, 1 cup	140	21	5	2	3.5	Low	ψ
imitation, nonsoy, 1 cup	112	12.9	3.9	0	4.9	ND	⊘
plain, soymilk, Silk, 1 cup	100	7	7	1	4	Low	ψψψ
unsweetened, soymilk, Silk, 1 cup	90	3	7	1	4	Low	ψψψ
vanilla, soymilk, Silk, 1 cup	100	9	6	1	3.5	Low	ψψψ

Food	Cal	Net Carb	Protein	Fiber	Total Fat	Glycemic Load	Advice
nonfat, 1 cup	86	12	8.4	0	0.4	Low	♈♈♈
reduced-fat, 2% milkfat, 1 cup	122	11.4	8.1	0	4.8	Low	♈♈
whole, 1 cup	146	11	7.9	0	7.9	Low	♈♈
Yogurt, 6 oz							
chocolate, nonfat milk	190	38	6	2	0	Low	⊗
frozen yogurt (*see* Desserts)							
fruit variety, nonfat	160	32.3	7.5	0	0.3	Low	⊗
fruit, low-fat	173	32.4	7.4	0	1.8	Low	⊗
plain, low-fat	107	12	8.9	0	2.6	Low	♈♈
plain, skim milk	95	13.1	9.7	0	0.3	Low	♈♈♈
plain, whole milk	104	7.9	5.9	0	5.5	Low	♈♈
soy yogurt (*see also* Legumes)							
Silk	160	28	4	1	2	Med.	♈
Stonyfield O'Soy	170	29	7	4	2	Med.	♈
Whole Soy	150	26	5	1	2.5	Med.	♈
vanilla or lemon flavor, nonfat milk, sweetened w/low-calorie sweetener	73	12.8	6.6	0	0.3	Low	♈
vanilla, low-fat	144	23.5	8.4	0	2.1	Low	⊗

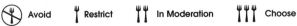

⊗ Avoid   ♈ Restrict   ♈♈ In Moderation   ♈♈♈ Choose

Desserts

I'M SURE BY NOW I DON'T NEED TO TELL YOU ALL THE REASONS TO avoid sugar. Besides being addictive for many people, having the worst possible metabolic effects, depressing the immune system, and, in recent studies, being linked with increased risk for heart disease and certain kinds of cancers, it also makes you fat. Really fat.

But you already knew that. The question is how to enjoy sweets with a minimum of damage. So I've included this section, which, although it lists many foods I'd never eat on a regular basis, contains some that are not so bad if you don't overdo them. Truth be told, even the worst of the lot can be eaten once in a while if you really only indulge on special occasions and adhere to the recommended portions. Part of the problem with these foods is that they taste so darn good that no one ever sticks to the suggested serving size. My ratings are going to assume that you do—if you don't, all bets are off.

In keeping with my "instinct" rule for rating foods that were on the borderline, I never recommend foods that I know to be sweetened primarily with fructose or high-fructose corn syrup, or any known to be loaded with trans-fats (animal crackers, for example).

You don't have to completely give up sweets and desserts when you're eating low-carb. You just have to be conscious of what you're eating, and how *much* you're really eating.

DESSERTS

Food	Cal	Net Carb	Protein	Fiber	Total Fat	Glycemic Load	Advice
Cake, 1 piece							
angelfood	72	15.8	1.7	0.4	0.2	Med.	
banana bread	196	32.1	2.6	0.7	6.3	High	
cheesecake	257	20.1	4.4	0.3	18	ND	
cheesecake, prepared from mix	271	33.3	5.5	1.9	12.6	ND	
chocolate w/chocolate frosting	235	33.1	2.6	1.8	10.5	Med.	
chocolate, no frosting	340	49.2	5	1.5	14.4	ND	
fruitcake	139	24.9	1.3	1.6	3.9	Med.	
gingerbread	263	36.4	2.9	ND	12.1	ND	
pineapple upside-down	367	57.2	4	0.9	13.9	ND	
pound	116	14.5	1.7	0.1	6	Low	
shortcake, 1 oz	98	13.8	1.7	ND	4	Low	
sponge	110	23	2.1	0.2	1	Med.	
white, no frosting	264	41.7	4	0.6	9.2	ND	
yellow w/chocolate frosting	243	34.3	2.4	1.2	11.1	Med.	
yellow w/vanilla frosting	239	37.4	2.2	0.2	9.3	Med.	
yellow, no frosting	245	35.5	3.6	0.5	9.9	ND	

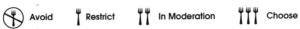

 Avoid   Restrict   In Moderation   Choose

Food	Cal	Net Carb	Protein	Fiber	Total Fat	Glycemic Load	Advice
Cookies							
animal crackers, 1 box (2 oz)	254	41.6	3.9	0.6	7.9	ND	🍴
butter, fructose sweetened, Fifty 50, 4 cookies	160	19	2	1	8	ND	🍴
chocolate and vanilla sandwich, fructose sweetened, Estee, 3 cookies	170	26	2	0	6	ND	🍴
chocolate chip, 2 cookies	156	18.6	1.8	ND	9.1	ND	🍴
chocolate chip soft-baked mini cookies, Atkins Endulge, 6 cookies*	170	6	5	8	11	ND	🍴
chocolate chip, fructose sweetened, Fifty 50, 4 cookies	170	19	2	1	9	ND	🍴
chocolate-coated marshmallow, 3 cookies	164	25.6	1.6	0.8	6.6	ND	🍴
chocolate fudge cookies, Atkins Endulge, 2 cookies*	120	4	2	5	7	ND	🍴🍴
chocolate sandwich w/crème filling, 3 cookies	142	20.1	1.4	1	6.2	ND	🍴
chocolate wafers, 3 wafers	78	12.4	1.2	0.6	2.6	ND	🍴🍴
coconut macaroon, 1 2" cookie	97	16.9	0.9	0.4	3.1	ND	🍴🍴
coconut, fructose sweetened, Fifty 50, 4 cookies	160	17	2	1	10	ND	🍴
crème-filled wafers, sugar-free, Fifty 50, 6 wafers*	160	11	1	1	9	ND	🍴
fig bar, 1 3" bar	99	18.9	1.1	1.3	2.1	ND	🍴
fortune, 1 cookie	30	6.6	0.3	0.1	0.2	ND	🍴
fudge, 1 cookie	73	15.8	1.1	0.6	0.8	ND	🍴

*contains sugar alcohols

ND = No Data

Food	Cal	Net Carb	Protein	Fiber	Total Fat	Glycemic Load	Advice
fudge brownie cookies, fructose sweetened, Fifty 50, 4 cookies	170	19	2	1	8	ND	
gingersnap, 4 cookies	116	20.9	1.6	0.6	2.7	ND	
graham crackers, 4 squares	118	20.7	1.9	0.8	2.8	Med.	
ladyfingers, 3 cookies	120	19.4	3.5	0.3	3	ND	
lemon, fructose sweetened, Estee, 4 cookies	160	18	2	2	8	ND	
molasses cookies, 1 large	138	23.3	1.8	0.3	4.1	ND	
oatmeal, 1 large	112	16.5	1.6	0.7	4.5	Low	
oatmeal raisin, 1 2-1/2" cookie	65	10.3	1	ND	2.4	Low	
oatmeal raisin, fructose sweetened, Estee, 4 cookies	160	20	2	1	7	ND	
peanut butter, 1 3" cookie	95	11.8	1.8	ND	4.8	ND	
peanut butter sandwich, 3 cookies	201	26.8	3.7	0.8	8.9	ND	
peanut butter sandwich, fructose sweetened, Estee, 3 cookies	190	24	4	1	8	ND	
pecan shortbread, 2 2" cookies	152	15.8	1.4	0.5	9.1	Low	
shortbread, 3 squares	120	15.1	1.5	0.4	5.8	Low	
sugar, 1 3" cookie	66	8.2	0.8	0.2	3.3	ND	
sugar-free, Sorbee, 1 cookie*	110	6	3	0	7	ND	
vanilla sandwich w/crème filling, 2 oval cookies	145	21.1	1.4	0.5	6	ND	

 Avoid   Restrict   In Moderation   Choose

Food	Cal	Net Carb	Protein	Fiber	Total Fat	Glycemic Load	Advice
vanilla wafers, 3 cookies	85	12.4	0.8	0.4	3.5	Low	🍴
vanilla, fructose sweetened, Estee, 4 cookies	160	20	2	1	7	ND	🚫
Frozen Desserts							
frozen yogurt, 1/2 cup							
Ben & Jerry's, Cherry Garcia	170	32	4	0	3	ND	🚫
Ben & Jerry's, chocolate fudge brownie	190	35	5	1	2.5	ND	🚫
Breyers Carb Smart, 4g net carbs, vanilla*	90	4	3	4	4.5	ND	🍴🍴🍴
Edy's, Heath toffee crunch	120	18	2	ND	4	ND	🍴
Edy's, vanilla	100	17	2	ND	2.5	ND	🍴
Haagen-Dazs, vanilla	200	31	8	0	4.5	ND	🚫
fruit ices, 1/2 cup unless noted							
ices, Rosati the Original Italian Water Ice, blue raspberry, 1 cup	150	32	1	0	0	ND	🚫
sherbet, Breyers, rainbow	130	27	1	0	1.5	ND	🚫
sherbet, Edy's, rainbow	130	29	1	ND	1	ND	🚫
sorbet, Breyers Carb Smart, 0g net carbs, chocolate*	70	0	2	2	4.5	ND	🍴🍴🍴
sorbet, Edy's Whole Fruit, blueberry	130	32	0	ND	0	ND	🚫
sorbet, Edy's Whole Fruit, tropical	150	38	0	ND	0	ND	🚫
sorbet, Haagen-Dazs, mango	120	30	0	1	0	ND	🚫

*contains sugar alcohols

Food	Cal	Net Carb	Protein	Fiber	Total Fat	Glycemic Load	Advice
Whole Fruit bar variety pack, Edy's, 1 small bar	60	13	0	ND	0	ND	⅋⅋
Whole Fruit bar, no sugar added, Edy's, variety pack, 1 small bar	30	8	0	ND	0	ND	⅋⅋⅋
ice cream, 1/2 cup							
chocolate, Breyers	150	16	3	1	8	Low	⅋
chocolate, Haagen-Dazs	270	21	5	1	18	Med.	⊘
chocolate, light, Breyers	140	19	4	1	5	Low	⅋
chocolate, low-carb, Atkins Endulge*	140	3	2	5	12	ND	⅋⅋⅋
chocolate, low-carb, Ben & Jerry's Carb Karma*	150	4	4	5	12	ND	⅋⅋⅋
chocolate, low-carb, Breyers Carb Smart, 4g net carbs*	130	4	2	3	10	ND	⅋⅋⅋
chocolate, low-carb, Edy's Carb Benefit*	150	3	2	7	10	ND	⅋⅋⅋
chocolate, no sugar added, Ben & Jerry's, New York Super Fudge Chunk*	220	5	4	5	18	ND	⊘
strawberry, Breyers	120	15	2	0	6	Low	⅋
strawberry, Haagen-Dazs	250	22	4	1	16	Med.	⊘
strawberry, no sugar added, Ben & Jerry's*	150	5	2	3	9	ND	⅋⅋
vanilla, Breyers	140	15	3	0	8	Low	⅋
vanilla, Haagen-Dazs	270	21	5	0	18	Med.	⊘
vanilla, soft-serve	191	18.5	3.5	0.6	11.2	Med.	⊘

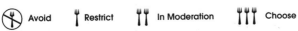

 Avoid   Restrict   In Moderation   ⅋⅋⅋ Choose

Food	Cal	Net Carb	Protein	Fiber	Total Fat	Glycemic Load	Advice
vanilla, light, Ben & Jerry's	160	19	4	0	7	Low	
vanilla, light, Breyers, natural vanilla	110	17	3	0	3	Low	
vanilla, light, Edy's Grand	100	15	3	ND	3.5	Low	
vanilla, low-carb, Atkins Endulge*	140	3	2	4	12	ND	
vanilla, low-carb, Ben & Jerry's Carb Karma, vanilla swiss almond*	170	2	5	4	15	ND	
vanilla, low-carb, Breyers Carb Smart, 0g net carbs*	130	0	5	3	9	ND	
vanilla, low-carb, Edy's Carb Benefit, vanilla bean*	140	4	2	6	9	ND	
vanilla, no sugar added, Breyers*	100	12	3	0	4.5	ND	
ice cream cones, 1 serving							
cake	17	3.1	0.3	0.1	0.3	ND	
sugar	40	8.2	0.8	0.2	0.4	ND	
waffle cone	121	22	2.4	0.9	2	ND	
ice cream singles and Popsicles, 1 serving							
chocolate chip cookie sandwich, Good Humor	290	40	3	1	13	ND	
chocolate fudge bars, low-carb, Atkins Endulge*	130	2	2	5	11	ND	
Creamsicle	110	20	1	0	3	ND	
Creamsicle, no sugar added*	25	5	1	0	0	ND	
Eskimo Pie Bar	166	12.3	2.1	0	12.1	ND	

*contains sugar alcohols

Food	Cal	Net Carb	Protein	Fiber	Total Fat	Glycemic Load	Advice
Fudgsicle	90	16	3	1	1.5	ND	
Fudgsicle, no sugar added, 2 pops*	90	15	3	1	1	ND	⍭
milk chocolate–covered ice cream bar, Good Humor	180	15	2	0	13	ND	
Klondike Bar	280	24	3	0	19	ND	
vanilla fudge swirl bars, low-carb, Atkins Endulge*	180	3	2	4	16	ND	⍭
vanilla sandwich, Good Humor	160	25	3	0	6	ND	
soy-based frozen desserts, nondairy, 1/2 cup							
low-carb, Carb Escapes, butter pecan ice cream*	150	6	2	9	12	Low	⍭
low-carb, Carb Escapes, chocolate peanut butter ice cream*	170	7	3	10	13	Low	⍭
low-carb, Carb Escapes, white mousse ice cream*	110	7	1	9	7	Low	⍭
low-carb, Carb Escapes, fudge bar, 1*	80	5	2	6	5	Low	⍭⍭
low-carb, Carb Escapes, vanilla bar, 1*	120	4	2	6	9	Low	⍭
Organic Soy Delicious, chocolate velvet ice cream	130	21	2	2	4	High	
Organic Soy Delicious, old-fashioned vanilla ice cream	120	19	2	5	4	High	
Organic Soy Delicious, strawberry ice cream	130	22	2	1	4	High	
Purely Decadent Soy Delicious, chocolate obsession	210	31	2	5	9	High	

 Avoid ⍭ Restrict ⍭⍭ In Moderation ⍭⍭⍭ Choose

Food	Cal	Net Carb	Protein	Fiber	Total Fat	Glycemic Load	Advice
Purely Decadent Soy Delicious, purely vanilla	170	23	1	6	8	High	🚫
It's Soy Delicious Fruit Sweetened Pints, awesome chocolate	130	23	2	1	3	High	🚫
It's Soy Delicious Fruit Sweetened Pints, green tea	110	22	2	2	1.5	High	🚫
It's Soy Delicious Fruit Sweetened Pints, vanilla	130	24	2	1	3	High	🚫
Soy Delicious Li'l Buddies, chocolate sandwich, 1 serving	150	25	3	3	4.5	High	🚫
Soy Delicious Li'l Buddies, vanilla sandwich, 1 serving	160	25	3	3	4.5	High	🚫
Mixes							
baking mix, **Atkins**, low-carb, 1/4 cup mix	80	3	13	5	0.5	ND	🍴🍴🍴
cake mix, no sugar, Sweet 'N Low, 1/3 cup mix*	160	21	3	1	3	ND	🚫
frosting, white, mix, no sugar, Sweet 'N Low, 2 tbsp	60	10	0	0	3	ND	🍴🍴
low-carb, chocolate chip cookie mix, **Atkins**, 2 2" cookies*	70	6	3	4	1	ND	🍴🍴🍴
Pastries							
brownies, 1, 2" square	112	12.1	1.5	ND	7	ND	🍴
cinnamon sweet roll, 1 roll	109	16.8	1.6	ND	4	Low	🍴
coffeecake, cinnamon crumb, 1 piece	263	28.1	4.3	1.3	14.7	Med.	🚫
éclair, 1 éclair	262	23.6	6.4	0.6	15.7	ND	🚫
strudel, apple, 1 piece	195	27.6	2.3	1.6	8	Med.	🚫

*contains sugar alcohols

Food	Cal	Net Carb	Protein	Fiber	Total Fat	Glycemic Load	Advice
Pie, 1 piece							
apple	411	57.5	3.7	ND	19.4	ND	
banana cream	387	46.4	6.3	1	19.6	ND	
blueberry	360	49.2	4	ND	17.5	ND	
Boston cream	232	38.2	2.2	1.3	7.8	ND	
cherry	486	69.3	5	ND	22	ND	
chocolate crème	301	31.3	2.6	2	19.2	ND	
chocolate mousse	247	28.1	3.3	ND	14.6	ND	
coconut cream	259	26.3	2.6	0.5	16.5	ND	
coconut custard	270	29.5	6.1	1.9	13.7	ND	
lemon meringue	362	49.7	4.8	ND	16.4	ND	
pecan	503	63.7	6	ND	27.1	ND	
pumpkin	316	40.9	7	ND	14.4	ND	
Puddings, 1/2 cup							
prepared from dry mix w/whole milk							
chocolate	169	26.5	4.6	1.1	4.5	Med.	
rice pudding	160	27.2	4.4	0.1	3.7	Med.	
tapioca	152	25.6	3.7	0	3.8	ND	

 Avoid   Restrict   In Moderation   Choose

Food	Cal	Net Carb	Protein	Fiber	Total Fat	Glycemic Load	Advice
vanilla	157	26.1	4	0.1	4.1	Med.	🍴
ready-to-eat							
chocolate, 1 snack size (4 oz)	157	24.9	3.1	1.1	4.5	ND	🍴
rice pudding, 1 serving (5 oz)	231	31.1	2.8	0.1	10.7	ND	🍴
tapioca, 1 snack size (4 oz)	134	21.8	2.3	0.1	4.2	ND	🍴
vanilla, 1 snack size (4 oz)	146	24.8	2.6	0	4.1	ND	🍴

Fast Food

I FIRST BECAME INTIMATELY FAMILIAR WITH FAST FOOD RESTAURANTS when I relocated from New York to Los Angeles and drove cross-country with my three dogs. Before that, I could count on one hand the number of times I had been inside a McDonald's and still have a couple of fingers left over. Not after that trip. I learned the hard way how to do damage control when fast food is all that's available, and now, thanks to the influence of my sixteen-year-old niece and nephew and my girlfriend Anja's teenage boy, I am a more frequent visitor to fast food restaurants than I ever thought I'd be.

And they've gotten marginally better. I'm still not a fan, but at least it's possible to navigate the minefield without committing nutritional suicide. Burger chains like Burger King and McDonald's now serve an array of salads; at many restaurants you can dump the bread from any entrée; and there's even an opportunity for damage control at Domino's, with medium crunchy thin-crust pizza. And Subway has recently become Atkins-friendly, though even in pre-Atkins days they had a pretty decent Mediterranean Chicken salad. Other sandwich chains, too, have heeded the low-carb call with fillings served in wraps or lower-carb flat breads.

Three caveats for eating at fast food restaurants are: lose the bread, watch portion sizes (twelve-inch sandwiches are obscenely high in calories), and never, under any circumstances, give in to the ridiculous notion that you simply must order french fries and a shake.

FAST FOOD

Food	Cal	Net Carb	Protein	Fiber	Total Fat	Advice
Burger King						
breakfast menu						
Croissan'wich w/egg & cheese	320	23	12	<1	19	
Croissan'wich w/sausage, egg & cheese	520	23	19	1	39	
Croissan'wich w/bacon, egg & cheese	360	24	15	<1	22	
Croissan'wich w/ham, egg & cheese	360	24	18	<1	20	
French Toast Sticks, 5 sticks	390	44	7	2	20	
hash brown rounds, 1 serving	230	21	2	2	15	
dessert menu						
Nestlè Toll House Cookies, 1 serving	440	68	5	0	16	
Dutch Apple Pie, 1 pie	340	51	2	1	14	
Hershey's Sundae Pie, 1 pie	300	30	3	1	18	
drinks (*see* Beverages)						
ICEE Coca Cola, 1 medium	450	113	0	0	0	
ICEE Cherry, 1 medium	450	113	0	0	0	
sandwiches and entrees						
BK Fish Fillet Sandwich	520	42	18	2	30	
BK Veggie (w/regular mayo)	380	42	14	4	16	
cheeseburger	350	30	19	1	17	

ND = No Data

Food	Cal	Net Carb	Protein	Fiber	Total Fat	Advice
chicken tenders, 5 pc	210	12	14	<1	12	
Chicken Whopper Sandwich	570	44	38	4	25	
hamburger	310	29	17	1	13	
Low-Carb Angus Steak Burger	280	4	25	<1	18	
Low-Carb Angus Bacon & Cheese Steak Burger	420	6	33	<1	29	
Original Chicken Sandwich	560	49	25	3	28	
Original Whopper	700	48	31	4	42	
Original Whopper w/cheese	800	49	35	4	49	
salads						
Fire-Grilled Chicken Caesar Salad	190	8	25	1	7	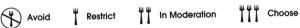
Fire-Grilled Chicken Garden Salad	210	11	26	2	7	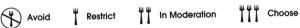
Fire-Grilled Shrimp Caesar Salad	180	7	19	2	10	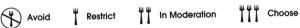
Fire-Grilled Shrimp Garden Salad	200	9	20	3	10	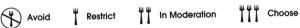
side garden salad	20	3	1	<1	0	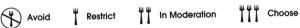
salad dressings, 1 serving						
Creamy Garlic Caesar	130	7	2	0	11	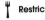
croutons	90	14	2	0	3	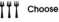
Garden Ranch	120	7	<1	0	10	

 Avoid   Restrict   In Moderation   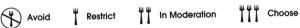 Choose

Food	Cal	Net Carb	Protein	Fiber	Total Fat	Advice
Hidden Valley Ranch, fat-free	35	7	0	0	0	🍴🍴
Sweet Onion Vinaigrette	100	8	0	0	8	🍴🍴
Tomato Balsamic Vinaigrette	110	9	0	0	9	🍴🍴
sides						
chili, 1 serving	190	12	13	5	8	🍴🍴
french fries, 1 medium	360	42	4	4	18	🚫
onion rings, 1 medium	320	37	4	3	16	🚫

Domino's Pizza

12" Medium Classic Hand-Tossed Pizza, 1 slice

Food	Cal	Net Carb	Protein	Fiber	Total Fat	Advice
America's Favorite Feast	257	27	10	2	11.5	🚫
Bacon Cheeseburger Feast	273	26	12	2	13	🚫
Barbecue Feast	252	30	11	1	10	🚫
beef	225	26	9	2	9	🚫
cheese	186	27	7	1	5.5	🚫
Deluxe Feast	234	27	9	2	9.5	🚫
ExtravaganZZa Feast	289	28	13	2	14	🚫
green pepper, onion, and mushroom	191	27	8	2	5.5	🚫
ham	198	27	9	1	6	🚫
ham and pineapple	200	27	9	2	6	🚫

Food	Cal	Net Carb	Protein	Fiber	Total Fat	Advice
Hawaiian Feast	223	28	10	2	8	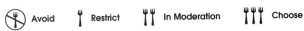
MeatZZa Feast	281	27	13	2	13.5	
pepperoni	223	26	9	2	9	
pepperoni and sausage	255	26	10	2	11.5	
Pepperoni Feast	265	26	11	2	12.5	
sausage	231	26	9	2	9.5	
Vegi Feast	218	27	9	2	8	
12" Medium Crunchy Thin-Crust Pizza, 1 slice						
America's Favorite Feast	208	14	8	1	13.5	
Bacon Cheeseburger Feast	224	13	10	1	14.5	
Barbecue Feast	203	16	8	1	11.5	
beef	175	13	7	1	10.5	
cheese	137	13	5	1	7	
Deluxe Feast	185	14	7	1	11.5	
ExtravaganZZa Feast	240	15	11	1	15.5	
green pepper, onion, and mushroom	142	14	6	1	7.5	
ham	148	13	7	1	7.5	
ham and pineapple	150	14	7	1	7.5	

 Avoid   Restrict   In Moderation   Choose

Food	Cal	Net Carb	Protein	Fiber	Total Fat	Advice
Hawaiian Feast	174	15	8	1	9.5	🍴🍴
MeatZZa Feast	232	14	11	1	15	🍴
pepperoni	174	13	7	1	10.5	🍴🍴
pepperoni and sausage	206	13	8	1	13.5	🍴
Pepperoni Feast	216	13	9	1	14	🍴
sausage	181	13	7	1	11	🍴🍴
Vegi Feast	168	14	7	1	9.5	🍴🍴
12" Medium Ultimate Deep Dish Pizza, 1 slice						
America's Favorite Feast	309	27	12	2	17	🚫
Bacon Cheeseburger Feast	325	26	14	2	18.5	🚫
Barbecue Feast	304	30	12	2	15	🚫
beef	277	26	11	2	14.5	🚫
cheese	238	26	9	2	11	🚫
Deluxe Feast	287	27	11	2	15	🚫
ExtravaganZZa Feast	341	28	14	2	19.5	🚫
green pepper, onion, and mushroom	244	28	9	2	11	🚫
ham	250	26	11	2	11.5	🚫
ham and pineapple	252	28	10	2	11.5	🚫
Hawaiian Feast	275	28	12	2	13	🚫

Food	Cal	Net Carb	Protein	Fiber	Total Fat	Advice
MeatZZa Feast	333	27	14	2	19	
pepperoni	275	26	11	2	14	
pepperoni and sausage	307	27	12	2	17	
Pepperoni Feast	317	27	13	2	17.5	
sausage	283	27	11	2	15	
Vegi Feast	270	28	11	2	13.5	
buffalo wings and condiments, 1 serving						
barbeque buffalo wings	50	2	6	0	2.5	
blue cheese dipping sauce	223	2	1	0	23.5	
Buffalo Chicken Kickers	47	3	4	0	2	
hot buffalo wings	45	1	5	0	2.5	
hot dipping sauce	15	4	0	0	0	
ranch dipping sauce	197	2	1	0	20.5	
side dishes, 1 serving						
breadsticks	115	12	2	0	6.3	
cheesy bread	123	13	4	0	6.5	
cinna stix	123	14	2	1	6.1	
garlic sauce	440	0	0	0	49	

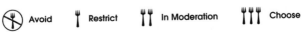

 Avoid   Restrict   In Moderation   Choose

Food	Cal	Net Carb	Protein	Fiber	Total Fat	Advice
marinara dipping sauce	25	5	1	0	0.2	🍴🍴
sweet icing	250	57	0	0	2.5	🍴

McDonald's

breakfast menu, 1 serving

Food	Cal	Net Carb	Protein	Fiber	Total Fat	Advice
bacon, egg, and cheese biscuit	430	30	18	1	26	🍴
Bacon, Egg & Cheese McGriddles	440	42	19	1	21	🍴
Egg McMuffin	300	26	18	2	12	🍴
hotcakes (w/2 pats of margarine and syrup)	600	104	9	0	17	🍴
sausage biscuit w/egg	490	30	16	1	33	🍴
Sausage, Egg & Cheese McGriddles	550	42	20	1	33	🍴
Sausage McGriddles	420	41	11	1	23	🍴
Sausage McMuffin w/Egg	250	27	20	2	28	🍴
warm cinnamon roll	510	77	8	4	23	🍴

chicken meals

Food	Cal	Net Carb	Protein	Fiber	Total Fat	Advice
Chicken McNuggets, 6 pc	250	15	15	0	15	🍴
Chicken Selects Premium Breast Strips, 5 pc	630	47	38	0	32	🍴

desserts/sweets, 1 serving

Food	Cal	Net Carb	Protein	Fiber	Total Fat	Advice
Baked Apple Pie	260	33	3	<1	13	🍴
Fruit 'n Yogurt Parfait	160	29	4	<1	2	🍴
Hot Caramel Sundae, 1 sundae	340	51	8	1	12	🍴

Food	Cal	Net Carb	Protein	Fiber	Total Fat	Advice
M&M McFlurry, 12 fl oz cup	630	89	16	1	23	
McDonaldland Chocolate Chip Cookies, 1 package	280	36	3	1	14	
McDonaldland Cookies, 1 package	230	37	3	1	8	
Oreo McFlurry, 12 fl oz cup	570	81	15	<1	20	
Strawberry Sundae, 1 sundae	290	49	7	<1	7	
vanilla reduced-fat ice cream cone, 1 cone	150	23	4	0	4.5	
french fries						
1 medium	350	40	5	4	17	
milkshakes						
Chocolate Triple Thick Shake, 16 fl oz cup	580	93	15	1	17	
Strawberry Triple Thick Shake, 16 fl oz cup	560	88	14	<1	16	
Vanilla Triple Thick Shake, 16 fl oz cup	470	89	14	0	16	
salads						
Crispy Chicken Caesar Salad	310	17	23	3	16	⅂⅂
Crispy Chicken Bacon Ranch Salad	350	17	26	3	19	⅂⅂
Fiesta Salad (w/o sour cream and salsa)	360	15	21	4	22	
Grilled Chicken Bacon Ranch Salad	250	6	31	3	10	⅂⅂
Grilled Chicken Caesar Salad	200	6	29	3	6	⅂⅂⅂
Grilled Chicken California Cobb Salad	370	17	27	3	21	⅂

 Avoid    Restrict   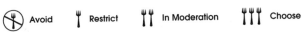 In Moderation   Choose

Food	Cal	Net Carb	Protein	Fiber	Total Fat	Advice
side salad	15	2	1	1	0	♈♈♈
salad dressings, 1 packet						
butter garlic croutons	50	8	1	0	1.5	⊘
Newman's Own Cobb Dressing	120	9	1	0	9	♈
Newman's Own Creamy Caesar Dressing	190	4	2	0	18	♈
Newman's Own Low-Fat Balsamic Vinaigrette	40	4	0	0	3	♈♈♈
Newman's Own Ranch Dressing	170	9	1	0	15	♈
Newman's Own Salsa	30	6	1	1	0	♈♈♈
sandwiches, 1 serving						
Big Mac	600	46	25	4	33	⊘
cheeseburger	330	34	15	2	14	⊘
Chicken McGrill	400	34	27	3	16	⊘
Crispy Chicken	510	44	22	3	26	⊘
Filet-O-Fish	410	40	15	1	20	⊘
hamburger	280	34	12	2	10	⊘
Quarter Pounder	430	35	23	3	21	⊘
Quarter Pounder w/Cheese	540	36	29	3	29	⊘

Pizza Hut

6" Personal Pan Pizza, 1 slice						
cheese	160	17	7	1	7	♈

Food	Cal	Net Carb	Protein	Fiber	Total Fat	Advice
chicken supreme	160	18	8	1	6	Restrict
meat lover's	200	17	9	1	10	Restrict
pepperoni	170	17	7	1	8	Restrict
pepperoni lover's	200	17	9	1	10	Restrict
quartered ham	150	17	7	1	6	Restrict
sausage lover's	190	17	8	1	10	Restrict
super supreme	200	18	9	1	10	In Moderation
supreme	190	18	8	1	9	In Moderation
veggie lover's	150	18	6	1	6	In Moderation
12" Medium Fit 'n Delicious, 1 slice						
diced chicken, red onion, and green pepper	170	21	10	2	4.5	Restrict
diced chicken, mushroom, and jalapeno	170	20	10	2	5	In Moderation
green pepper, red onion, and diced red tomato	150	22	6	2	4	In Moderation
ham, pineapple, and diced red tomato	160	22	8	2	4	In Moderation
ham, red onion, and mushroom	160	20	8	2	4.5	Restrict
tomato, mushroom, and jalapeno	150	20	6	2	4	Restrict
12" Medium Hand-Tossed Pizza, 1 slice						
cheese	240	28	12	2	8	Avoid

 Avoid   Restrict   In Moderation   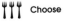 Choose

Food	Cal	Net Carb	Protein	Fiber	Total Fat	Advice
chicken supreme	230	28	14	2	6	🍴
meat lover's	300	27	15	2	13	🍴
pepperoni	250	27	12	2	9	🍴
pepperoni lover's	300	28	15	2	13	🍴
quartered ham	220	27	12	2	6	🍴
sausage lover's	280	28	13	2	12	🍴
super supreme	300	29	15	2	13	🍴
supreme	270	28	13	2	11	🍴
veggie lover's	220	29	10	2	6	🍴
12" Medium Pan Pizza, 1 slice						
cheese	280	28	11	1	13	🍴
chicken supreme	280	28	13	2	12	🍴
meat lover's	340	27	15	2	19	🍴
pepperoni	290	28	11	1	15	🍴
pepperoni lover's	340	27	15	2	19	🍴
quartered ham	260	28	11	1	11	🍴
sausage lover's	330	27	13	2	17	🍴
super supreme	340	28	14	2	18	🍴
supreme	320	28	13	2	16	🍴

Food	Cal	Net Carb	Protein	Fiber	Total Fat	Advice
veggie lover's	260	28	10	2	12	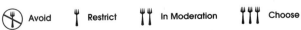
12" Medium Thin 'n Crispy Pizza, 1 slice						
cheese	200	20	10	1	8	
chicken supreme	200	21	12	1	7	
meat lover's	270	19	13	2	14	
pepperoni	210	20	10	1	10	
pepperoni lover's	260	19	13	2	14	
quartered ham	180	20	9	1	6	
sausage lover's	240	19	11	2	13	
super supreme	260	21	13	2	13	
supreme	240	20	11	2	11	
veggie lover's	180	21	8	2	7	
appetizers/sides						
breadsticks, 1 serving	150	19	4	1	6	
breadstick dipping sauce, 3 oz	50	9	1	2	0	
cheese breadsticks, 1 serving	200	20	7	1	10	
hot wings, 2 pieces	110	1	11	0	6	
marinara dipping sauce, 1 serving	45	7	2	2	0	

Avoid   Restrict   In Moderation   Choose

Food	Cal	Net Carb	Protein	Fiber	Total Fat	Advice
mild wings, 2 pieces	110	1	11	0	7	🍴🍴
wing blue cheese dipping sauce, 1.5 oz	230	2	2	0	24	🍴
wing ranch dipping sauce, 1.5 oz	210	4	<1	0	22	🍴
desserts						
Apple Dessert Pizza	260	52	4	1	3.5	🍴
Cherry Dessert Pizza	240	46	4	1	3.5	🍴
cinnamon sticks, 2 pieces	170	26	4	1	5	🍴
white icing dipping cup, 2 oz	190	46	0	0	0	🍴
P'ZONES						
classic, 1/2 serving	610	68	33	3	21	🍴
meat lover's, 1/2 serving	680	67	38	3	28	🍴

Subway

6" subs						
Cheese Steak	360	42	24	5	10	🍴
Chipotle Southwest Cheese Steak	440	44	24	5	19	🍴
Classic Tuna	430	42	20	4	19	🍴
Cold Cut Combo	410	42	21	4	17	🍴
Dijon Turkey Breast, Ham, and Bacon Melt	470	43	26	5	21	🍴
Ham	290	42	18	4	5	🍴

Food	Cal	Net Carb	Protein	Fiber	Total Fat	Advice
Honey Mustard Ham	310	49	19	5	5	
Italian BMT	450	43	23	4	21	
Meatball Marinara	500	47	23	5	22	
Oven-Roasted Chicken Breast	330	42	24	5	5	
Roast Beef	290	41	19	4	5	
Savory Turkey Breast	280	42	18	4	4.5	
Subway Seafood Sensation	380	47	16	5	13	
Sweet Onion Chicken Teriyaki	370	54	26	5	5	
Turkey Breast, Ham, and Bacon Melt	380	43	25	4	12	
Turkey Breast, Ham, and Roast Beef	320	43	24	4	6	
Veggie Delite	230	40	9	4	3	
Atkins-friendly wraps						
Chicken Bacon Ranch	480	8	40	11	27	
Mediterranean Chicken	350	8	36	9	18	
Turkey Bacon Melt	430	10	32	12	25	
Turkey Breast and Ham	390	10	32	9	23	
breakfasts, omelettes, and french toast						
bacon and egg	240	2	20	0	17	

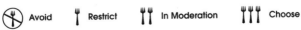

Avoid   Restrict   In Moderation   Choose

Food	Cal	Net Carb	Protein	Fiber	Total Fat	Advice
cheese and egg	240	2	19	0	17	🍴🍴
french toast w/syrup	350	55	14	2	8	🚫
ham and egg	230	2	21	0	14	🍴🍴
steak and egg	250	2	24	1	15	🍴🍴
vegetable and egg	210	3	17	1	14	🍴🍴🍴
western egg	220	3	19	1	14	🍴🍴
breakfast sandwiches on 6" Italian or wheat bread						
bacon and egg	450	39	28	3	19	🚫
cheese and egg	440	39	27	3	19	🚫
ham and egg	430	39	29	3	17	🚫
steak and egg	460	39	33	4	18	🚫
vegetable and egg	410	40	25	4	16	🚫
western egg	430	40	27	4	17	🚫
breakfast sandwiches on deli round rolls						
bacon and egg	320	31	15	3	15	🚫
cheese and egg	320	31	14	3	15	🚫
ham and egg	310	31	16	3	13	🚫
steak and egg	330	32	19	3	14	🚫
vegetable and egg	290	33	12	3	12	🚫

Food	Cal	Net Carb	Protein	Fiber	Total Fat	Advice
western egg	300	33	14	3	12	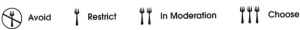
deli-style sandwiches						
classic tuna	300	33	13	3	13	
ham	210	32	11	3	4	
roast beef	220	32	13	3	4.5	
savory turkey breast	210	33	13	3	3.5	
promotional/regional subs, 6"						
Baja Chicken	350	40	26	5	9	
Baja Pork	530	45	38	5	21	
Barbecue Pulled Pork	440	49	31	4	13	
BBQ Rib Patty	420	43	20	4	19	
Buffalo Chicken	400	41	25	4	15	
Carne Asada	420	41	36	4	11	
Chicken Fajita	510	43	32	6	21	
Gardenburger	390	56	19	10	7	
Lloyd's BBQ Chicken	310	47	16	5	6	
Mediterranean Chicken	440	41	30	5	16	
Pastrami	570	44	32	5	29	

 Avoid Restrict In Moderation Choose
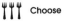

Food	Cal	Net Carb	Protein	Fiber	Total Fat	Advice
Spicy Italian	480	41	21	4	25	🚫🍴
Steak Fajita	500	45	29	7	21	🚫🍴
Veggi-Max	390	49	24	7	8	🚫🍴
salads						
Classic Club	390	9	37	4	21	🍴🍴
Garden Fresh	60	6	3	5	1	🍴🍴🍴
Grilled Chicken and Spinach	420	5	38	5	26	🍴🍴
Mediterranean Chicken	170	6	22	5	4.5	🍴🍴🍴
salad dressings and condiments						
Atkins Honey Mustard	200	1	1	0	22	🍴
bacon bits	50	0	5	0	4.5	🍴🍴
croutons	70	8	1	0	3	🚫🍴
diced eggs	45	0	4	0	3	🍴🍴🍴
garlic almonds	80	1	3	2	7	🍴🍴🍴
Greek Vinaigrette	200	3	1	0	21	🍴
Kraft Fat-Free Italian	35	7	1	0	0	🍴
Kraft Ranch	200	0.5	1	0.5	22	🚫🍴
Red Wine Vinaigrette	80	17	1	0	1	🍴🍴🍴

Food	Cal	Net Carb	Protein	Fiber	Total Fat	Advice
smoothies, Fruizle Express, 1 small						
Berry Lishus	110	27	1	1	0	
Sunrise Refresher	120	28	1	1	0	
Pineapple Delight	130	32	1	1	0	
Peach Pizzazz	100	26	0	0	0	
soup, 1 cup serving						
cheese w/ham and bacon	240	16	8	1	15	
chicken and dumpling	130	15	7	1	4.5	
chili con carne	240	15	15	8	10	
cream of broccoli	130	13	5	2	6	
cream of potato w/bacon	200	19	4	2	11	
golden broccoli and cheese	180	14	5	2	11	
New England-style clam chowder	110	15	5	1	3.5	
roasted chicken noodle	60	6	6	1	1.5	
Spanish-style chicken w/rice	90	12	5	1	2	
tomato garden vegetable w/rotini	100	18	3	2	0.5	
sweets and cookies, 1 serving						
apple pie	245	36	0	1	10	
Atkins-Friendly Double Chocolate cookies	100	7	2	5	6	

 Avoid   Restrict   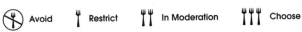 In Moderation   Choose

Food	Cal	Net Carb	Protein	Fiber	Total Fat	Advice
chocolate chip cookies	210	29	2	1	10	🍴⊘
Fruit Roll-Up	50	12	0	0	1	🍴
sugar cookies	230	28	2	0	12	🍴⊘
white macadamia nut cookies	220	27	2	1	11	🍴⊘
Taco Bell						
beef dishes, 1 serving						
Burrito Supreme	440	44	18	7	18	🍴⊘
Chalupa Supreme	390	28	14	3	24	🍴⊘
Chili Cheese Burrito	390	37	16	3	18	🍴⊘
crunchy taco	170	10	8	3	10	🍴🍴🍴
Fiesta Burrito	370	45	18	3	12	🍴⊘
Fresco-Style crunchy taco, low-fat	150	11	7	3	7	🍴🍴🍴
Fresco-Style soft taco, low-fat	190	19	9	3	8	🍴🍴
Gordita Supreme	310	27	14	3	16	🍴⊘
Grilled Stuft Burrito	730	69	28	10	33	🍴⊘
soft taco	210	19	10	2	10	🍴🍴
Soft Taco Supreme	260	19	11	3	14	🍴⊘
Taco Supreme	220	11	9	3	14	🍴🍴

Food	Cal	Net Carb	Protein	Fiber	Total Fat	Advice
chicken dishes, 1 serving						
Burrito Supreme	410	45	21	5	14	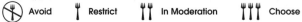
Chalupa Supreme	370	29	17	1	20	
Fiesta Burrito	370	44	16	4	13	
Fresco-Style Burrito Supreme, low-fat	350	44	19	6	8	
Fresco-Style Fiesta Burrito, low-fat	350	45	16	4	9	
Fresco-Style Ranchero Chicken Soft Taco, low-fat	170	20	12	2	4.5	
Gordita Supreme	290	26	17	2	12	
Grilled Stuft Burrito	680	69	35	7	26	
Ranchero Chicken soft taco	270	19	13	2	15	
Soft Taco Supreme	230	20	15	1	10	
vegetarian burritos, 1 serving						
7-Layer Burrito	530	56	18	10	21	
bean burritos	370	47	14	8	10	
Fresco-Style bean burrito, low-fat	350	47	13	9	8	
nachos and sides, 1 serving						
cinnamon twists	160	28	<1	0	5	
nachos	320	31	5	2	19	
Nachos BellGrande	780	68	20	12	43	

 Avoid   Restrict   In Moderation   Choose

Food	Cal	Net Carb	Protein	Fiber	Total Fat	Advice
Nachos Supreme	450	35	13	7	26	🍴
Pintos 'n Cheese	180	14	10	6	7	🍴
Mexican rice	210	20	6	3	10	🍴
salads, 1 serving						
Express Taco Salad w/chips	620	47	27	13	31	🍴
Fiesta Taco Salad	870	65	32	15	48	🍴
Fiesta Taco Salad, no shell	500	29	25	13	26	🍴
Southwest Steak Bowl	700	60	30	13	32	🍴
Zesty Chicken Border Bowl	730	53	23	12	42	🍴
Zesty Chicken Border Bowl, no dressing	500	48	22	12	19	🍴
specialties, 1 serving						
Cheese Quesadilla	490	36	19	3	28	🍴
Chicken Quesadilla	540	37	28	3	30	🍴
Enchirito, beef	380	29	19	6	18	🍴
Enchirito, chicken	350	28	23	5	14	🍴
Fresco-Style Enchirito, beef, low-fat	270	28	13	7	9	🍴
Fresco-Style Enchirito, chicken, low-fat	250	29	16	5	5	🍴
Fresco-style Tostada, low-fat	200	22	8	8	6	🍴
Mexican Pizza	550	39	21	7	31	🍴

Food	Cal	Net Carb	Protein	Fiber	Total Fat	Advice
MexiMelt	290	20	15	3	16	⍦
Tostada	250	22	11	7	10	⍦
Wendy's						
desserts						
Frosty, 1 medium	430	74	10	0	11	Ⓨ
Frosty, 1 small	330	56	8	0	8	Ⓨ
sandwiches and entrees, 1 serving						
Big Bacon Classic	580	42	33	3	29	Ⓨ
chicken nuggets, 5 pc	220	13	10	0	14	⍦⍦
Classic Single Hamburger	410	35	25	2	19	Ⓨ
Homestyle Chicken Fillet Sandwich	540	55	29	2	22	Ⓨ
Homestyle Chicken Strips, 3 pc	410	33	28	0	18	Ⓨ
Spicy Chicken Fillet Sandwich	510	55	29	2	19	Ⓨ
Ultimate Chicken Grill Sandwich	360	42	31	2	7	Ⓨ
salads, 1 serving						
Caesar side salad	70	1	6	1	4.5	⍦⍦
Chicken BLT Salad	360	6	34	4	19	⍦
Homestyle Chicken Strips Salad	450	29	29	5	22	Ⓨ
Mandarin Chicken Salad	190	14	22	3	3	⍦⍦⍦

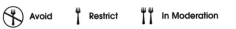

Ⓨ Avoid   ⍦ Restrict   ⍦⍦ In Moderation   ⍦⍦⍦ Choose

Food	Cal	Net Carb	Protein	Fiber	Total Fat	Advice
side salad	35	4	2	3	0	🍴🍴🍴
Spring Mix Salad	180	7	11	5	11	🍴🍴🍴
Taco Supremo Salad	360	21	27	8	16	🍴🍴
salad dressings and condiments, 1 serving						
barbecue sauce	40	10	1	0	0	🍴🍴🍴
Caesar dressing	150	1	1	0	16	🍴
Creamy Ranch dressing	230	5	1	0	23	⊘
Creamy Tangy Sauce, 1/2 oz	70	1	0	0	7	🍴🍴
crispy noodles	60	10	1	0	2	⊘
Deli Honey Mustard Sauce	170	6	0	0	16	⊘
fat-free French-style dressing	80	19	0	0	0	⊘
Honey Mustard dressing	280	11	1	0	26	⊘
House Vinaigrette dressing	190	8	0	0	18	⊘
low-fat Honey Mustard	110	21	0	0	3	⊘
Heartland Ranch Sauce	200	1	0	0	21	⊘
Homestyle Garlic croutons	70	9	1	0	2.5	⊘
honey mustard sauce	130	6	0	0	12	🍴🍴
honey-roasted pecans	130	3	2	2	13	🍴🍴
Oriental Sesame dressing	250	19	1	0	19	⊘

Food	Cal	Net Carb	Protein	Fiber	Total Fat	Advice
reduced-fat Creamy Ranch dressing	100	5	1	1	8	In Moderation
roasted almonds	130	2	5	2	11	Choose
salsa	30	6	1	0	0	Choose
Spicey Southwest Chipotle Sauce	140	5	0	0	13	In Moderation
sweet & sour sauce	45	12	0	0	0	Avoid
sides, 1 serving						
baked potato w/bacon and cheese	560	60	16	7	25	Avoid
baked potato w/broccoli and cheese	440	61	10	9	15	Avoid
baked potato, plain	270	54	7	7	0	Avoid
baked potato w/sour cream and chives	340	55	8	7	6	Avoid
chili, 1 small	200	16	17	5	5	In Moderation
chili, 1 large	300	24	25	7	7	Avoid
french fries, 1 kid's meal	250	32	3	4	11	Avoid
french fries, 1 medium	390	50	4	6	17	Avoid
taco chips	220	25	3	2	11	Avoid

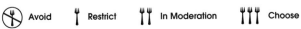

Avoid   Restrict   In Moderation   Choose

Fats and Oils

FATS COME IN MANY FORMS, AND THE DIFFERENT FORMS HAVE varying effects on your diet.

Bad fats are *damaged* fats. Fats can be damaged by high heat or chemical processing. The worst of all are trans-fats, found in baked goods, french fries, cookies, crackers, and margarine. My advice: don't eat them...ever.

Omega-6s—found in vegetable oils, corn oils, sunflower, safflower, and the like—are quite pro-inflammatory. Oils that are extremely high in omega-6s were not recommended in this section.

Saturated fats from natural, whole food sources are not necessarily bad. Just be sure to balance your saturated fat intake with omega-3s (from fish and flaxseed) and omega-9s (from macadamia nut oil and olive oil).

Rating fats and oils is difficult because you have to consider what the fat or oil is being used for, as well as how it was processed. Omega-3 fats, rightly acclaimed for health benefits, should never be used for cooking. Peanut oil has a high smoke point (good), but also a very high level of omega-6s (not good). High-oleic sunflower oil has lots of healthy omega-9s (good), but is highly refined (not good).

For salads, try flaxseed oil, hempseed oil, or one of the cooking oils—macadamia nut oil, olive oil, coconut oil, etc. For cooking, try macadamia nut oil, which has a great ratio of omega-6 to omega-3 fats, tons of omega-9s, and a high smoke point. Extra virgin olive oil, good old-fashioned butter, and coconut oil—probably my favorite—are all great. Refined oils like corn, safflower, sunflower, and soybean are far too high in omega-6s and are highly processed. I'm not a fan of canola oil either, because it is highly refined.

For more information on oils, consult *The Hamptons Diet*, by Dr. Fred Pescatore; chapter 5 is a great consumer guide.

FATS AND OILS						
Food	**Cal**	**Net Carb**	**Protein**	**Fiber**	**Total Fat**	**Advice**
Animal Fat, 1 tbsp unless noted						
bacon grease, 1 tsp	39	0	0	0	4.4	⅋
beef tallow	115	0	0	0	12.8	⅋⅋
chicken fat	115	0	0	0	12.8	⅋⅋
cod liver oil	123	0	0	0	13.6	⅋⅋⅋
duck fat	115	0	0	0	12.8	⅋⅋
goose fat	115	0	0	0	12.8	⅋⅋
herring oil	123	0	0	0	13.6	⅋⅋
lard	115	0	0	0	12.8	⅋⅋
mutton tallow	115	0	0	0	12.8	⅋
salmon oil	123	0	0	0	13.6	⅋⅋⅋
sardine oil	123	0	0	0	13.6	⅋⅋⅋
turkey fat	115	0	0	0	12.8	⅋⅋
Butter, Margarine, and Alternatives						
butter, 1 tsp						
butter	34	0	0	0	3.8	⅋⅋⅋
butter, whipped	22	0	0	0	2.5	⅋⅋⅋

 Avoid 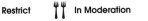 Restrict   In Moderation   Choose

Food	Cal	Net Carb	Protein	Fiber	Total Fat	Advice
clarified butter (ghee)	45	0	0	0	5	🍴🍴🍴
margarine						
Country Crock plus calcium, 1 tbsp	50	0	0	0	5	🚫
I Can't Believe It's Not Butter stick, 1 tbsp	90	0	0	0	10	🚫
I Can't Believe It's Not Butter stick, light, 1 tbsp	50	0	0	0	6	🚫
spread, 20% fat, 1 tsp	9	0	0	0	1	🚫
spread, 40% fat, 1 tsp	17	0	0	0	1.9	🚫
spread, 60% fat, 1 tsp	26	0	0	0	2.9	🚫
spread, 70% soybean oil, 1 tbsp	87	0.2	0	0	9.7	🚫
stick, 80% fat, corn and soybean oils, 1 tbsp	99	0.3	0	0	11	🚫
stick, regular, 1 tsp	34	0	0	0	3.8	🚫
tub, regular 80% fat, 1 tsp	34	0	0	0	3.8	🚫
soft spreads, 1 tbsp unless noted						
Benecol	70	0	0	0	8	🍴🍴
Benecol Light	45	0	0	0	5	🍴🍴
Brummel & Brown made w/yogurt	45	0	0	0	5	🍴🍴
Country Crock plus yogurt (no trans-fat)	40	0	0	0	4	🍴🍴
Fleischmann's made w/olive oil	70	0	0	0	8	🚫
Fleischmann's original	70	0	0	0	8	🚫

ND = No Data

Food	Cal	Net Carb	Protein	Fiber	Total Fat	Advice
I Can't Believe It's Not Butter spray, 1-1/2 sprays	0	0	0	0	0	🍴🍴
I Can't Believe It's Not Butter tub (no trans-fat)	80	0	0	0	9	🍴🍴
I Can't Believe It's Not Butter tub light (no trans-fat)	50	0	0	0	5	🍴🍴
I Can't Believe It's Not Butter w/calcium (no trans-fat)	50	0	0	0	5	🍴🍴
Parkay squeeze	70	0	0	0	8	⊘
Promise	80	0	0	0	8	⊘
Promise light	45	0	0	0	5	⊘
Smart Balance	80	0	0	0	9	⊘
Smart Balance light	45	0	0	0	5	⊘
Smart Balance Omega Plus	80	0	0	0	9	🍴🍴
Smart Beat	20	0	0	0	2	🍴
Spectrum Naturals spread	80	0	0	0	10	🍴🍴🍴
Oils, 1 tbsp						
almond oil	120	0	0	0	13.6	🍴🍴🍴
apricot kernel oil	120	0	0	0	13.6	🍴🍴
avocado oil	124	0	0	0	14	🍴🍴🍴
canola oil	124	0	0	0	14	⊘
coconut oil	117	0	0	0	13.6	🍴🍴🍴

 Avoid   Restrict   In Moderation   🍴🍴🍴 Choose

Food	Cal	Net Carb	Protein	Fiber	Total Fat	Advice
corn oil	120	0	0	0	13.6	⊘
cottonseed oil	120	0	0	0	13.6	⊘
flaxseed oil	120	0	0	0	13.6	🍴🍴🍴
grapeseed oil	120	0	0	0	13.6	⊘
hazelnut oil	120	0	0	0	13.6	🍴
hemp seed oil	126	0	0.5	0	14	🍴🍴🍴
macadamia nut oil	120	0	0	0	14	🍴🍴🍴
olive oil	119	0	0	0	13.5	🍴🍴🍴
palm kernel oil	117	0	0	0	13.6	🍴🍴
peanut oil	119	0	0	0	13.5	🍴🍴
perilla oil	125	0	0	0	14	🍴🍴🍴
rice bran oil	120	0	0	0	13.6	🍴🍴
safflower oil	120	0	0	0	13.6	⊘
sesame oil	120	0	0	0	13.6	🍴🍴
soybean oil	120	0	0	0	13.6	⊘
sunflower oil	124	0	0	0	14	⊘
teaseed oil	120	0	0	0	13.6	🍴🍴🍴
walnut oil	120	0	0	0	13.6	🍴

Food	Cal	Net Carb	Protein	Fiber	Total Fat	Advice
wheat germ oil	120	0	0	0	13.6	Restrict

Other Fats

Food	Cal	Net Carb	Protein	Fiber	Total Fat	Advice
avocado, raw, 1/2 cup, sliced	117	1.3	1.5	4.9	10.7	Choose
coconut meat						
dried, creamed, 1 oz	194	6.1	1.5	ND	19.6	Choose
dried, sweetened, 1 oz	134	12.3	0.9	1.2	9.1	Restrict
dried, unsweetened, 1 oz	187	2.1	2	4.6	18.3	Choose
raw, 1 piece (2"x2"x1/2")	159	2.9	1.5	4	15.1	Choose
half and half	20	0.7	0.4	0	1.7	Choose
heavy cream	52	0.4	0.3	0	5.6	Choose
olives, pickled, green, 4 tbsp	48	0.2	0.3	1.1	5.1	Choose
olives, ripe, canned, 4 tbsp (1/4 cup)	39	1	0.3	1.1	3.6	Choose

Shortening, 1 tbsp

Food	Cal	Net Carb	Protein	Fiber	Total Fat	Advice
for baking						
soybean	113	0	0	0	12.8	Avoid
palm	113	0	0	0	12.8	Avoid
cottonseed	113	0	0	0	12.8	Avoid
coconut	113	0	0	0	12.8	Choose

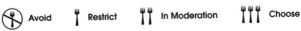

Avoid   Restrict   In Moderation   Choose

Food	Cal	Net Carb	Protein	Fiber	Total Fat	Advice
for frying						
beef tallow	115	0	0	0	12.8	♈♈♈
cottonseed	115	0	0	0	12.8	⊘
spreads, 1 tbsp						
mayonnaise	100	0	0	0	11	♈
mayonnaise, low-calorie	32	2.2	0	0	2.7	♈♈
mayonnaise, made w/tofu	48	0.4	0.9	0.2	4.7	♈♈
sour cream	26	0.5	0.4	0	2.5	♈♈♈
sour cream, fat-free, Kraft	15	2.4	0.8	0	0.2	♈♈♈
sour cream, reduced-fat	20	0.6	0.4	0	1.8	♈♈♈

Fruits

"EAT YOUR FRUITS AND VEGETABLES" HAS BEEN REPEATED SO OFTEN that it's become a ho-hum platitude. Remember, though, that from a blood-sugar point of view these two classes of food are not exactly equal. If I had to choose one, it would be no contest: vegetables are the clear winner.

That's because fruit—wonderful though it is—has a lot of sugar, and can play havoc with both blood sugar and insulin. For this reason, some controlled-carb programs don't allow fruit at all during the first phase of weight loss. Almost all the nutrients found in fruits are obtainable in vegetables, and with substantially less impact on blood sugar. That said, no low-carb program needs to be completely without fruit. But it's a good idea to set limits, especially in the beginning.

Choose fruits that have a lower glycemic load—berries, for example. Melons are good as well: they're high in water, low in calories, and pretty low in sugar. Apples are a great source of fiber, and are also one of the main dietary sources of boron, a trace mineral that is not only important for bone health, but can also be used to treat fatigue.

Even fruits with a relatively high glycemic impact (grapes, for example) can be worked into a good controlled-carb program; compared with such glycemic nightmares as pasta and bread, they're relatively innocuous as long as you don't go overboard. And when I'm craving sweets—especially in maintenance phase—I freeze some grapes and snack on about fifteen of them. Frozen berries—with a little half and half or whipped cream—are another delight. Either will beat the heck out of a box of cookies.

FRUITS

Food	Cal	Net Carb	Protein	Fiber	Total Fat	Glycemic Load	Advice
apples							
dried, uncooked, 1 cup	209	49.2	0.8	7.5	0.3	Med.	⛟
dried, uncooked, 1 ring	16	3.6	0.1	0.6	0	Low	⛟⛟⛟
raw, w/skin, 1 medium	72	15.8	0.4	3.3	0.2	Low	⛟⛟⛟
w/o skin, boiled, 1 cup	91	19.2	0.4	4.1	0.6	Low	⛟⛟
applesauce, sweetened, 1/2 cup	97	24	0.3	1.6	0.3	ND	🚫
applesauce, unsweetened, 1/2 cup	58	12.4	0.2	1.5	0	ND	⛟
apricots							
canned, in juice w/skin, 1 apricot half w/liquid	17	3.8	0.2	0.6	0	ND	⛟⛟⛟
canned, light syrup w/skin, 1 apricot half w/liquid	25	6	0.2	0.6	0	Low	⛟⛟
canned, in water w/skin, 1 apricot half w/liquid	10	1.7	0.3	0.6	0.1	ND	⛟⛟⛟
dried, uncooked, 1/4 cup	78	18	1.1	2.4	0.2	Low	⛟⛟
dried, uncooked, 1 half	8	1.9	0.1	0.3	0	Low	⛟⛟⛟
raw, 1 apricot	17	3.2	0.5	0.7	0.1	Low	⛟⛟⛟
avocados, raw, all commercial varieties, 1/4 cup	60	0.7	0.8	2.5	5.5	ND	⛟⛟⛟
bananas, raw, 1 medium	105	23.9	1.3	3.1	0.4	Med.	⛟
blackberries, canned, heavy syrup, 1/2 cup	118	25.2	1.7	4.4	0.2	ND	🚫

Food	Cal	Net Carb	Protein	Fiber	Total Fat	Glycemic Load	Advice
blackberries, frozen, unsweetened, 1 cup	97	16.2	1.8	7.5	0.7	ND	👍👍
blackberries, raw, 1 cup	62	6.2	2	7.6	0.7	ND	👍👍👍
blueberries, frozen, sweetened, 1/2 cup	93	23	0.5	2.5	0.2	ND	👍
blueberries, frozen, unsweetened, 1 cup	79	14.7	0.7	4.2	1	ND	👍👍👍
blueberries, raw, 1 cup	83	17.5	1.1	3.5	0.5	ND	👍👍👍
boysenberries, canned, heavy syrup, 1/2 cup	113	25.2	1.3	3.4	0.2	ND	🚫
boysenberries, frozen, unsweetened, 1 cup	66	9.1	1.5	7	0.3	ND	👍👍👍
cantaloupe, raw, 1 cup	54	11.7	1.3	1.4	0.3	ND	👍👍👍
casaba, raw, 1 cup	48	9.7	1.9	1.5	0.2	ND	👍👍👍
cherries, 1 cup unless noted							
maraschino, canned, drained (100 grams)	165	38.8	0.2	3.2	0.2	ND	🚫
sour, canned, light syrup	189	46.6	1.9	2	0.3	Med.	🚫
sour, canned, in water	88	19.1	1.9	2.7	0.2	Low	👍👍
sour, frozen, unsweetened	71	14.6	1.4	2.5	0.7	Low	👍👍👍
sour, raw, 1 cup, pitted	78	16.4	1.6	2.5	0.5	Low	👍👍👍
sweet, canned in juice, pitted	135	30.7	2.3	3.8	0.1	Low	🚫
sweet, canned in light syrup, pitted	169	39.8	1.5	3.8	0.4	Low	🚫
sweet, canned in water, pitted	114	25.5	1.9	3.7	0.3	Low	👍

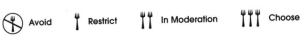

 Avoid   Restrict   In Moderation   Choose

Food	Cal	Net Carb	Protein	Fiber	Total Fat	Glycemic Load	Advice
sweet, frozen, sweetened	231	52.5	3	5.4	0.3	Med.	🚫🍴
sweet, raw, pitted, 1/2 cup	46	10.1	0.8	1.5	0.2	Low	🚫🍴
sweet, raw, 1 cherry	4	1	0.1	0.1	0	Low	🍴🍴🍴
cranberries, dried, sweetened, 1/4 cup	92	23	0	1.7	0.4	ND	🍴🍴
cranberries, raw, 1 cup, whole	44	7.2	0.4	4.4	0.1	ND	🍴🍴🍴
cranberry sauce, canned, sweetened, 1 slice (1/2" thick, 8 slices per can)	86	21.6	0.1	0.6	0.1	ND	🍴🍴
currants, European black, raw, 1/2 cup	36	8.5	0.5	5.1	0.3	ND	🍴🍴🍴
currants, red and white, raw, 1 cup	63	10.7	1.6	4.8	0.2	ND	🍴🍴🍴
dates, Deglet Noor, 1/2 cup, pitted, chopped	251	59.7	2.2	7.1	0.4	ND	🚫🍴
dates, Medjool, 1 date, pitted	66	16.4	0.4	1.6	0	ND	🍴
elderberries, raw, 1/2 cup	53	8.3	0.5	5.1	0.4	ND	🍴🍴🍴
fig, raw, 1 medium	37	8.2	0.4	1.4	0.2	ND	🍴🍴
figs, dried, uncooked, 1/2 cup	186	40.3	2.5	7.3	0.7	High	🚫🍴
fruit cocktail, light syrup, 1/2 cup	69	16.9	0.5	1.2	0.1	Low	🚫🍴
fruit cocktail, in juice, 1/2 cup	55	12.9	0.6	1.2	0	Low	🍴
fruit cocktail, in water, 1/2 cup	38	8.9	0.5	1.2	0.1	Low	🍴🍴
gooseberries, canned, light syrup, 1/2 cup	92	20.6	0.8	3	0.3	ND	🚫🍴
gooseberries, raw, 1/2 cup	33	4.4	0.7	3.2	0.4	ND	🍴🍴🍴

Food	Cal	Net Carb	Protein	Fiber	Total Fat	Glycemic Load	Advice
grapefruit							
raw, pink, red and white, 1/2 medium	41	8.9	0.8	1.4	0.1	Low	⚟⚟⚟
canned, in juice, 1 cup	92	21.9	1.7	1	0.2	ND	⚟
canned, light syrup, 1 cup	152	38.2	1.4	1	0.3	ND	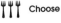
canned, in water, 1 cup	88	21.3	1.4	1	0.2	ND	⚟
grapes, American-type, raw, 1 cup	62	15	0.6	0.8	0.3	Low	⚟⚟⚟
grapes, red or green, European-type, raw, 1 cup, seedless	110	27.6	1.2	1.4	0.3	Med.	⚟
groundcherries (cape-gooseberries or poha), raw, 1 cup	74	15.7	2.7	ND	1	ND	⚟⚟⚟
guavas, common, raw, 1 cup	84	10.7	1.4	8.9	1	ND	⚟⚟⚟
guavas, strawberry, raw, 1/2 cup	84	15	0.7	6.6	0.8	ND	⚟
honeydew, raw, 1 cup	61	14.1	0.9	1.4	0.2	ND	⚟⚟⚟
kiwi fruit (Chinese gooseberries), fresh, raw, 1/2 cup	54	10.4	1	2.7	0.5	Med.	⚟⚟⚟
kumquats, raw, 1 fruit	13	1.8	0.4	1.2	0.2	ND	⚟⚟⚟
lemons, raw, w/o peel, 1 wedge or slice	2	0.5	0.1	0.2	0	ND	⚟⚟⚟
limes, raw, 1 fruit	15	3.7	0.3	1.9	0.1	ND	⚟⚟⚟
litchis, dried, 1 fruit	7	1.7	0.1	0.1	0	Low	⚟⚟⚟
litchis, raw, 1/2 cup	63	15	0.8	1.3	0.4	Med.	⚟⚟

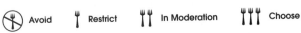

 Avoid   ⚟ Restrict   ⚟⚟ In Moderation   ⚟⚟⚟ Choose

Food	Cal	Net Carb	Protein	Fiber	Total Fat	Glycemic Load	Advice
mangos, raw, 1/2 cup, sliced	54	12.5	0.4	1.5	0.3	Med.	♟♟
mulberries, raw, 1 cup	60	11.4	2	2.4	0.6	ND	♟♟♟
nectarines, raw, 1 fruit, medium	60	12.1	1.4	2.3	0.4	ND	♟♟♟
oranges, raw, all commercial varieties, 1 medium	62	12.3	1.2	3.1	0.2	Low	♟♟♟
papayas, raw, 1 cup, cubed	55	11.2	0.9	2.5	0.2	Low	♟♟♟
passion-fruit, granadilla, purple, raw, 1 cup	229	30.7	5.2	24.5	1.7	ND	⊘
peaches							
canned in juice, 1/2 cup	55	12.8	0.8	1.6	0.1	Low	♟♟
canned in light syrup, 1/2 cup	68	16.6	0.6	1.7	0.1	Med.	♟
canned in water, 1 cup	59	11.7	1.1	3.2	0.2	ND	♟♟♟
dried, uncooked, 1/4 cup	95	21.5	1.5	3.3	0.3	ND	♟
frozen, sliced, sweetened, 1/2 cup	118	27.8	0.8	2.3	0.2	ND	⊘
raw, 1 fruit, medium	38	7.8	0.9	1.5	0.2	Low	♟♟♟
pears							
Asian, raw, 1 fruit	51	8.6	0.6	4.4	0.3	Low	♟♟♟
canned in juice, 1/2 cup	62	14	0.4	2	0.1	Med.	♟♟
canned in light syrup, 1/2 cup	72	17	0.3	2	0.1	Low	♟
canned in water, 1/2 cup	36	7.6	0.3	2	0.1	ND	♟♟
dried, uncooked, 1/2 cup	236	55.9	1.7	6.8	0.6	ND	⊘

Food	Cal	Net Carb	Protein	Fiber	Total Fat	Glycemic Load	Advice
raw, 1 fruit, medium	96	20.6	0.6	5.1	0.2	Low	
persimmons, Japanese, dried, 1 fruit	93	20.1	0.5	4.9	0.2	ND	
persimmons, Japanese, raw, 1 fruit (2-1/2" dia.)	118	25.2	1	6	0.3	ND	
persimmons, native, raw, 1 fruit	32	8.4	0.2	ND	0.1	ND	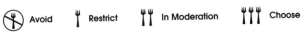
pineapple, 1/2 cup							
canned in juice	75	18.5	0.6	1	0.1	ND	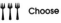
canned in juice, drained	55	13	0.5	1.2	0.1	ND	
canned in light syrup	65	16	0.5	1	0.2	ND	
canned in water	40	9.2	0.6	1	0.1	ND	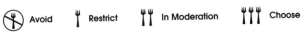
frozen, chunks, sweetened	106	26	0.5	1.4	0.1	Med.	
raw, all varieties, in chunks	37	8.7	0.4	1.1	0.1	Med.	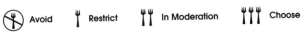
raw, extra-sweet variety, in chunks	40	9.4	0.4	1.1	0.1	Med.	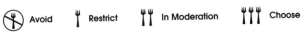
plantains, cooked, 1/2 cup, sliced	90	22.3	0.6	1.8	0.2	ND	
plantains, raw, 1 cup, sliced	90	22	1	1.7	0.3	ND	
plums							
canned in juice, 1/2 cup	73	18	0.7	1.1	0.1	ND	
canned in light syrup, 1/2 cup	80	19.3	0.5	1.2	0.2	ND	
canned in water, 1/2 cup	51	12.6	0.5	1.1	0	ND	

 Avoid   Restrict   In Moderation   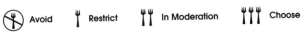 Choose

Food	Cal	Net Carb	Protein	Fiber	Total Fat	Glycemic Load	Advice
dried (prunes), stewed, 1/2 cup	133	31	1.2	3.8	0.2	Low	♀
dried (prunes), uncooked, 1/2 cup	204	48.3	1.9	6	0.3	Med.	⊘
raw, 1 fruit	30	6.6	0.5	0.9	0.2	Low	♀♀♀
pomegranates, raw, 1 fruit	105	25.5	1.5	0.9	0.5	ND	♀
prickly pears, raw, 1 fruit	42	6.2	0.8	3.7	0.5	ND	♀♀♀
prunes, canned, heavy syrup pack, 1/2 cup	123	28.1	1	4.4	0.2	Low	⊘
prunes, dehydrated, stewed, 1/2 cup	158	41.6	1.7	3.8	0.3	Med.	⊘
prunes, dehydrated, uncooked, 1/2 cup	224	58.8	2.4	6	0.5	Med.	⊘
quinces, raw, 1 fruit, w/o refuse	52	12.4	0.4	1.7	0.1	ND	♀♀♀
raisins, golden seedless, 1/4 cup, not packed	109	27.4	1.2	1.4	0.2	Med.	♀
raisins, seedless, 1/4 cup, not packed	108	27.4	1.1	1.3	0.2	Med.	♀
raspberries, canned, heavy syrup pack, 1 cup	233	51.4	2.1	8.4	0.3	ND	⊘
raspberries, frozen, sweetened, 1/2 cup	129	27.2	0.9	5.5	0.2	ND	⊘
raspberries, raw, 1 cup	64	6.7	1.5	8	0.8	ND	♀♀♀
rhubarb, frozen, cooked, w/sugar, 1 cup	278	70.1	0.9	4.8	0.1	ND	⊘
rhubarb, frozen, uncooked, 1 cup	29	4.5	0.8	2.5	0.2	ND	♀♀♀
rhubarb, raw, 1 cup, cubed	26	3.3	1.1	2.2	0.2	ND	♀♀♀
starfruit (carambola), raw, 1 cup, cubed	45	7	0.7	3.7	0.5	ND	♀♀♀

Food	Cal	Net Carb	Protein	Fiber	Total Fat	Glycemic Load	Advice
strawberries, frozen, unsweetened, 1 cup	77	15.6	1	4.6	0.2	Low	🍴🍴
strawberries, raw, 1 cup	46	8.2	1	2.9	0.4	Low	🍴🍴🍴
tamarinds, raw, 2 fruits	5	1.2	0.1	0.1	0	ND	🍴🍴🍴
tangerines (mandarin oranges)							
canned in juice, 1 cup	92	22.1	1.5	1.7	0.1	ND	🍴🍴
canned in juice, drained, 1 cup	72	15.5	1.4	2.3	0.1	ND	🍴🍴
canned in light syrup, 1 cup	154	39	1.1	1.8	0.3	ND	🚫
raw, 1 medium	37	7.5	0.5	1.9	0.2	ND	🍴🍴🍴
watermelon, raw, 1 cup, cubed	46	10.9	0.9	0.6	0.2	Low	🍴🍴🍴

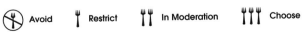

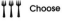 Avoid   Restrict   🍴🍴 In Moderation   🍴🍴🍴 Choose

Grains

A FREQUENT CRITICISM OF LOW-CARB DIETS IS THAT THEY'RE LOW IN fiber. The truth is, nearly all American diets are low in fiber. You can easily eat a ton of commercial cereal and bread—the standard high-carb diet—and still be consuming less than ten grams of fiber a day. You should be consuming thirty. The question is whether you'll get it from grains.

And the answer is...not if they're processed. The trick with grains is to get them as free from processing as possible. The food industry has made this devilishly difficult, confusing consumers with all manner of "wheat breads"—which are nothing more than white bread with a little brown sugar thrown in—and other whole-grain imposters.

Then there's the allergy problem. Grains—particularly wheat— are among the most allergenic substances on the planet. While they don't always induce full-blown allergies, they frequently provoke what's called a "food sensitivity reaction." This reaction can involve a host of symptoms from bloat to fatigue to headache to joint pain. Some of the top nutritionists in America have a very simple program when dealing with weird, unexplainable symptoms: cut out all dairy, wheat, and sugar.

That said, whole grains are not a bad thing (think steel-cut oats instead of instant oatmeal). Read nutrition labels for fiber content. I wouldn't consider any cereal that has less than five grams of fiber per serving, with minimal sugar. I've seen hot cereals from companies like LowCarb Success that have a whopping thirteen grams of fiber per serving. I grab these off the shelves whenever I'm traveling. You should too.

GRAINS						
Food	**Cal**	**Net Carb**	**Protein**	**Fiber**	**Total Fat**	**Glycemic Load**	**Advice**
Breads, 1 slice unless noted						
bagels, 1 serving						
cinnamon-raisin	323	62.4	11.6	2.7	2	High+	
egg	364	66.4	13.9	3	2.8	High+	
oat bran	280	54.6	11.8	4	1.3	High+	
original, low-carb, Thomas' Carb Counting	110	12	12	12	2.5	ND	
original, low-carb, Thomas' Carb Consider	150	18	11	6	2.5	ND	
plain	302	56.2	11.6	2.5	1.8	High+	
poppy	302	56.2	11.6	2.5	1.8	High+	
whole-wheat, low-carb, Thomas' Carb Counting	110	12	12	12	2.5	ND	
whole-wheat, low-carb, Thomas' Carb Consider	140	16	11	7	2.5	ND	
biscuits						
1 biscuit	93	12.4	1.8	0.4	4	ND	
low-carb, Atkins, 1 biscuit	25	1	4	3	0	ND	
low-fat, 1 biscuit	63	11.2	1.6	0.4	1.1	ND	
cornbread, 1 piece	188	27.5	4.3	1.4	6	ND	
English muffins						
1 plain muffin	134	24.7	4.4	1.5	1	Med.	

 Avoid   Restrict   In Moderation   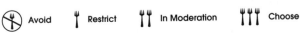 Choose

Food	Cal	Net Carb	Protein	Fiber	Total Fat	Glycemic Load	Advice
low-carb, Thomas' Carb Consider	100	14	7	9	1.5	ND	🍴
cinnamon-raisin	139	26.1	4.3	1.7	1.5	Med.	🚫🍴
whole-wheat	134	22.3	5.8	4.4	1.4	Med.	🚫🍴
loaf bread							
cracked wheat	65	11	2.2	1.4	1	Low	🍴
egg	115	18.2	3.8	0.9	2.4	ND	🚫🍴
French or sourdough	175	31.3	5.6	1.9	1.9	Med.	🚫🍴
Irish soda, 1 oz	82	15.2	1.9	0.7	1.4	ND	🍴
Italian	54	9.5	1.8	0.5	0.7	Low	🍴
multi-grain, low-carb, Arnold Carb Counting	60	6	5	3	1.5	Low	🍴🍴🍴
mixed grain	65	10.4	2.6	1.7	1	Low	🍴
oat bran	71	10.5	3.1	1.4	1.3	Low	🍴
oatmeal	73	12	2.3	1.1	1.2	ND	🍴
pita, white, 16-1/2" pita	165	32.1	5.5	1.3	0.7	Med.	🚫🍴
pita, whole-wheat, 16-1/2" pita	170	30.5	6.3	4.7	1.7	ND	🚫🍴
pumpernickel	65	10.7	2.3	1.7	0.8	Low	🍴
raisin	71	12.5	2.1	1.1	1.1	ND	🍴
rice bran	66	10.4	2.4	1.3	1.2	ND	🍴

*contains sugar alcohols

ND = No Data

Food	Cal	Net Carb	Protein	Fiber	Total Fat	Glycemic Load	Advice
rye	83	13.6	2.7	1.9	1.1	Low	
wheat	65	10.7	2.3	1.1	1	Low	
white	80	14.5	2.3	0.7	1	Med.	
whole-wheat	69	11	2.7	1.9	1.2	Low	
whole-wheat, low-carb, Arnold Carb Counting	60	6	4	4	1.5	Low	
whole-wheat, low-carb, Roman Meal Carb Aware*	60	6	5	2	1	Low	
whole-wheat, low-carb, Schmidt Carb Alert*	60	6	5	2	1	Low	
Breakfast Cereals							
All-Bran, 1/2 cup	78	12.6	3.8	9.6	1	Low	
Amaranth Flakes, 1 cup	134	23.4	5.9	3.6	2.7	High	
Atkins Banana Nut Harvest, 2/3 cup	100	5	12	6	2.5	ND	
Atkins Blueberry Bounty w/almonds, 2/3 cup	100	4	13	6	2	ND	
Atkins Crunchy Almond Crisp, 2/3 cup	100	3	15	5	1.5	ND	
Banana Nut Crunch, 1 cup	249	39.7	5	4	6.1	ND	
Basic 4, 1 cup	202	39.2	4.4	3.2	2.8	ND	
Blueberry Morning, 1-1/4 cup	211	41.3	3.6	2.1	2.5	ND	
Bran Flakes, 3/4 cup	96	18.8	2.8	5.3	0.7	Med.	
Carb Well High Protein, 3/4 cup	110	9	11	5	2	ND	

  Avoid   Restrict   In Moderation   Choose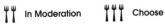

Food	Cal	Net Carb	Protein	Fiber	Total Fat	Glycemic Load	Advice
Cheerios							
regular, 1 cup	111	19.5	3.3	2.7	1.8	Med.	🍴
multi-grain, 1 cup	108	21.6	2.4	2.7	1.2	Med.	🍴
Chex							
corn, 1 cup	112	25.2	2.1	0.6	0.3	High	🍴
multi-bran, 1 cup	166	34.8	3.4	6.4	1.2	Med.	🍴
rice, 1-1/4 cup	117	26.4	1.9	0.3	0.3	High	🍴
wheat, 1 cup	104	21	3	3.3	0.6	ND	🍴
Cinnamon Grahams, 3/4 cup	113	24.8	1.5	1	0.8	ND	🍴
Corn Flakes, 1 cup	101	23	1.9	1.3	0	Med.	🍴
corn grits, cooked w/water, 1 cup	143	30.5	3.4	0.7	0.5	ND	🍴
Corn Pops, 1 cup	118	27.7	1.2	0.2	0.2	High	🍴
Cracklin' Oat Bran, 3/4 cup	225	32.9	4.6	6.4	8	Med.	🍴
Cream of Rice, cooked w/water, 1 cup	127	27.9	2.2	0.2	0.2	ND	🍴
Cream of Wheat, cooked w/water, 1 cup	149	30.1	4.4	1.4	0.6	High	🍴
Crispix, 1 cup	109	24.8	2	0.1	0.2	High	🍴
Crispy Brown Rice, 1 cup	124	25.2	2.3	2.3	1.1	ND	🍴
Farina, cooked w/water, 1 cup	112	23.7	3.3	0.7	0.2	ND	🍴
Fiber One, 1/2 cup	59	9.9	2.4	14.4	0.8	ND	🍴🍴🍴

Food	Cal	Net Carb	Protein	Fiber	Total Fat	Glycemic Load	Advice
Fruit & Fibre, 1 cup	212	36.6	3.9	5.3	3.1	ND	⊗
Golden Crisp, 3/4 cup	107	24.5	1.5	0	0.4	ND	⊗
Golden Grahams, 3/4 cup	112	24	1.5	0.9	1.1	Med.	⊗
Granola, 1/2 cup	299	27.1	9.1	5.2	14.9	ND	⊗
Granola, low-fat w/raisins, 2/3 cup	201	41.2	4.4	2.8	2.8	ND	⊗
Grape-Nuts, 1/2 cup	208	42.2	6.3	5	1.1	High+	⊗
Grape-Nuts Flakes, 3/4 cup	106	21	2.9	2.6	0.8	Med.	⊗
Great Grains, crunchy pecan, 2/3 cup	216	34.1	4.9	3.7	6.3	ND	⊗
Great Grains, raisin, date, and pecan, 2/3 cup	204	35.5	4.3	4	4.5	ND	⊗
Honey Bunches of Oats, 3/4 cup	118	23.1	2.1	1.5	1.7	ND	⊗
Honey Crunch Corn Flakes, 3/4 cup	117	25.1	2	1	1	Med.	⊗
hot cereal, low-carb, Carb Sense, Country Spice, 1/2 cup dry	170	3	12	12	7	ND	🍴🍴🍴
hot cereal, low-carb, Carb Sense, Hazelnut, 1/2 cup dry	190	3	12	12	9	ND	🍴🍴🍴
Just Right Fruit and Nut, 1 cup	201	42	3.9	2.9	1.8	High	⊗
Kix, 1-1/3 cup	113	24.9	1.8	0.9	0.6	ND	⊗
Mini-Wheats, apple cinnamon, 3/4 cup	182	39.4	4	4.7	1	High	⊗

⊗ Avoid   🍴 Restrict   🍴🍴 In Moderation   🍴🍴🍴 Choose

Food	Cal	Net Carb	Protein	Fiber	Total Fat	Glycemic Load	Advice
Mini-Wheats, frosted, 1 cup	173	35.9	5	5.1	0.8	High	
Mueslix, 2/3 cup	196	36.2	5	4	3	High	
Oat Bran, dry, 1/2 cup	73	9.8	3.4	2.9	1.6	Med.	
Oatmeal Squares, 1 cup	212	39.9	6.2	4	2.4	ND	
Oatmeal Squares, cinnamon, 1 cup	227	43.3	6.1	4.6	2.6	ND	
oatmeal, instant, apples and cinnamon, 1 packet prepared	130	23.8	2.7	2.7	1.5	Med.	
oatmeal, instant, maple and brown sugar, 1 packet prepared	157	28.3	3.7	2.8	2	Med.	
oats, 1 cup cooked	129	18.7	5.4	3.7	2.1	Low	
Product 19, 1 cup	100	23.9	2.3	1	0.4	ND	
Puffed Rice, 1 cup	54	12.1	1	0.2	0.1	Low	
Puffed Wheat, 1-1/4 cup	55	10.1	2.4	1.4	0.3	Low	
Raisin Bran, 1 cup	187	38.4	4.7	7.7	1.1	High	
Raisin Bran Crunch, 1 cup	188	41	3.2	4	1	High	
Raisin Nut Bran, 1 cup	209	36.4	5.2	5.1	4.4	High	
Rice Krispies, 1-1/4 cup	119	28.9	2.1	0.1	0.4	High	
Shredded Wheat, 2 biscuits	156	32.8	4.8	5.3	0.6	High	
Shredded Wheat 'N Bran, 1-1/4 cup	197	39.2	7.4	7.9	0.8	ND	
Smacks, 3/4 cup	104	23	1.7	1	0.5	Med.	

Food	Cal	Net Carb	Protein	Fiber	Total Fat	Glycemic Load	Advice
Smart Start, 1 cup	182	40.7	3.1	2.3	0.6	ND	Avoid
Special K, 1 cup	117	21.3	7	0.7	0.5	Med.	Avoid
Special K Red Berries, 1 cup	114	24	3.8	1	0.3	Med.	Avoid
Total, 3/4 cup	97	20.1	2.4	2.4	0.8	Med.	Avoid
wheat bran, 1 cup	125	12.6	9	24.8	2.5	Med.	Choose
Wheatena, cooked w/water, 1 cup	136	22.1	4.9	6.6	1.2	ND	Restrict
Wheaties, 1 cup	106	21.3	3	3	1	Med.	Avoid
Cooked Grains, 1/2 cup							
barley, pearled	97	10.7	1.8	3	0.4	Low	Restrict
buckwheat groats, roasted	78	14.5	2.9	2.3	0.5	Low	Restrict
bulgur	76	12.8	2.8	4.1	0.2	Low	Restrict
hominy, canned, white	60	9.7	1.2	2.1	0.8	Low	In Moderation
hominy, canned, yellow	58	9.4	1.2	2	0.7	Low	Restrict
millet	104	19.5	3.1	1.2	0.9	Med.	Avoid
oatbran	44	9.7	3.5	2.9	1	Low	In Moderation
quinoa	64	6.5	3	2	2	ND	In Moderation
Crackers (*see* Snacks)							

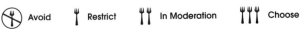

Avoid   Restrict   In Moderation   Choose

Food	Cal	Net Carb	Protein	Fiber	Total Fat	Glycemic Load	Advice
Doughnuts and Pastries, 1 serving							
breakfast bars							
Atkins Morning Start, apple crisp	170	2	11	6	9	ND	🍴🍴🍴
Atkins Morning Start, chocolate chip crisp	160	2	13	5	7	ND	🍴🍴🍴
Kellogg Mini's w/yogurt icing	160	31	2	1	3	ND	🍴
Nutri-Grain Twists and Cereal Bars	140	26	1	1	3	Med.	🍴
Quaker Oatmeal Breakfast Squares, brown sugar cinnamon	220	40	4	3	4	ND	🍴
Quaker Oatmeal Breakfast Squares, oatmeal raisin	220	39	4	4	4	ND	🍴
cinnamon danish	572	61.5	9.9	1.8	31.8	High+	🍴
cinnamon sweet roll, 1 roll	109	16.8	1.6	ND	4	Med.	🍴
coffeecake, cinnamon crumb, 1 piece	263	28.1	4.3	1.3	14.7	Med.	🍴
danish, cheese	266	25.7	5.7	0.7	15.6	High	🍴
danish, nut	280	28.4	4.6	1.3	16.4	High	🍴
doughnuts							
chocolate frosting	270	26.3	2.9	1.1	17.7	High	🍴
crème filling	307	24.8	5.4	0.7	20.8	Med.	🍴
jelly	289	32.4	5	0.8	15.9	High	🍴
plain	299	34.2	3.6	1.1	16.3	High	🍴

*contains sugar alcohols

Food	Cal	Net Carb	Protein	Fiber	Total Fat	Glycemic Load	Advice
French cruller, 1 cruller	169	23.9	1.3	0.5	7.5	ND	
French toast, 1 slice	149	16.3	5	ND	7	ND	
muffin, blueberry	465	76.2	9.2	4.4	10.9	High+	
muffin, corn	512	79.8	9.9	5.7	14.1	High+	
muffin, oatbran	454	73.4	11.8	7.7	12.4	High+	
strudel, apple, 1 piece	195	27.6	2.3	1.6	8	Med.	
toaster pastries, 1 pastry	204	35.9	2.4	1.1	5.3	High	
Pancakes and Waffles							
pancakes							
blueberry, 1 6" pancake	171	22.3	4.7	ND	7.1	Med.	
buttermilk, 1 6" pancake	175	22.1	5.2	ND	7.2	Med.	
low-carb, Atkins, 1/4 cup mix	80	3	13	3	1.5	ND	⫿⫿⫿
low-carb, Sweet 'N Low, 1/3 cup mix*	150	24	5	1	0	ND	
waffles							
7" round waffle	218	24.7	5.9	ND	10.6	Med.	
Kellogg's Eggo low-fat homestyle, 2 waffles	165	30.2	4.9	0.7	2.5	High	
Kellogg's Eggo low-fat Nutri-Grain, 2 waffles	142	25.6	4.4	2.6	2.2	Med.	
low-carb, Kellogg's, Eggo, 2 waffles	190	8	15	7	11	ND	⫿⫿⫿

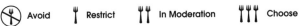

 Avoid   ⫿ Restrict   ⫿⫿ In Moderation   ⫿⫿⫿ Choose

Food	Cal	Net Carb	Protein	Fiber	Total Fat	Glycemic Load	Advice
low-carb, Thomas' Carb Consider, 1 waffle	110	11	6	6	5	ND	🍴🍴🍴
Pastas, 1 cup cooked unless noted							
chow mein noodles	237	24.1	3.8	1.8	13.8	ND	🍴
corn pasta	176	32.4	3.7	6.7	1	ND	🍴
couscous	176	34.3	6	2.2	0.3	High	🍴
egg and spinach noodles	211	35.1	8.1	3.7	2.5	ND	🍴
egg noodles	213	37.9	7.6	1.8	2.4	Med.	🍴
low-carb, Bella Vita, dry	160	10	28	8	1	ND	🍴🍴🍴
macaroni	189	36.3	6.4	1.7	0.9	Med.	🍴
soba noodles	113	24.4	5.8	ND	0.1	Med.	🍴
spaghetti	197	37.3	6.7	2.4	0.9	Med.	🍴
spinach spaghetti	182	36.6	6.4	ND	0.9	ND	🍴
vegetable macaroni	172	29.9	6.1	5.8	0.2	ND	🍴
whole-wheat macaroni	174	33.3	7.5	3.9	0.8	ND	🍴
whole-wheat spaghetti	174	30.9	7.5	6.3	0.8	Med.	🍴
Rice, 1 cup unless noted							
brown, long-grain	216	41.3	5	3.5	1.8	High	🍴
brown, medium-grain	218	42.3	4.5	3.5	1.6	High	🍴

Food	Cal	Net Carb	Protein	Fiber	Total Fat	Glycemic Load	Advice
white, long-grain	205	43.9	4.3	0.6	0.4	High	
white, long-grain, instant	162	34.1	3.4	1	0.3	High	
white, medium-grain	242	52.6	4.4	0.6	0.4	High	
white, short-grain	242	53.4	4.4	ND	0.4	High	
wild	166	32	6.5	3	0.6	High	
rice noodles	192	42	1.6	1.8	0.4	High	
Tortilla							
tortilla, 1 serving, 1 6" dia.	58	10.7	1.5	1.4	0.7	Low	In Moderation
low-carb, Atkins, 1 tortilla	100	5	7	6	5	ND	Choose
whole-wheat, 1 large tortilla	120	20	4	2	3	Low	Restrict
Wheat Products							
wheat germ, crude, 1/8 cup	52	5.6	3.3	1.9	1.4	ND	Choose
wheat gluten, seitan, White Wave, chicken-style, 1 piece	130	2	20	10	0	ND	Choose
wheat gluten, seitan, White Wave, traditional, 1 piece	140	2	31	1	1	ND	Choose

 Avoid    Restrict   In Moderation   Choose

Legumes

BEANS HAVE A LOT GOING FOR THEM, BUT THEIR TOP SELLING POINT is fiber. It's hard to think of a food that's higher in fiber, and, as you know, I'm a huge fan of high-fiber diets. That's the good news.

There are two potential problems with beans that are worth noting. The first has to do with their high carbohydrate content and the fact that some of them have relatively high glycemic ratings (baked beans, for example). The book *Atkins Diabetes Revolution* files kidney beans and dried peas under "eat in moderation," and puts black-eyed peas, dried lima beans, navy beans, and pinto beans on the "eat sparingly" list. I agree completely.

The other potential problem with beans stems from lectin sensitivity. Lectins are carbohydrate-linking proteins that can initiate a cascade of immune system responses when they bind themselves to cell surfaces along the gut wall or on arteries, glands, or organs. Some people are more susceptible to lectins than others, and the reactions vary widely; those found in kidney beans often result in the standard food-poisoning symptom, gastric upset.

If you've experienced sensitivity to the lectins in beans, you might want to try eliminating them altogether and see how you feel. Lectins may be deactivated by soaking, sprouting, cooking, or fermenting. Soaking legumes overnight, draining the water, rinsing the beans, and draining them again does seem to remove or deactivate many of the lectins.

LEGUMES

Food	Cal	Net Carb	Protein	Fiber	Total Fat	Glycemic Load	Advice
Beans and Legumes, cooked, 1/2 cup unless noted							
adzuki	147	20.1	8.7	8.4	0.1	ND	♟♟
baked beans, vegetarian, canned	118	19.7	6.1	6.4	0.6	Low	♟♟
baked beans, w/pork, canned	134	18.4	6.6	7	2	Low	♟♟
black	114	12.9	7.6	7.5	0.5	Low	♟♟♟
chickpeas	135	16.3	7.3	6.3	2.2	Low	♟♟♟
fava	94	12.1	6.5	4.6	0.4	ND	♟♟♟
french	114	13	6.3	8.3	0.7	ND	♟♟♟
great northern	105	12.5	7.4	6.2	0.4	ND	♟♟♟
hummus (chickpeas), 1 tbsp	23	1.2	1.1	0.8	1.3	Low	♟♟♟
hyacinth	114	20.1	7.9	N/A	0.6	ND	♟♟
kidney	113	14.6	7.7	5.7	0.5	Low	♟♟
lentils	115	12.2	9	7.8	0.4	Low	♟♟♟
lima beans	108	13.1	7.4	6.6	0.4	Low	♟♟♟
mothbeans	104	18.6	6.9	N/A	0.5	ND	♟♟
mung	106	11.7	7.1	7.7	0.4	Low	♟♟♟

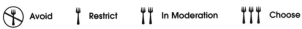

 Avoid   ♟ Restrict   ♟♟ In Moderation   ♟♟♟ Choose

Food	Cal	Net Carb	Protein	Fiber	Total Fat	Glycemic Load	Advice
mungo	95	10.8	6.8	5.8	0.5	Low	♟♟♟
navy, haricot	129	18.2	7.9	5.8	0.5	Low	♟♟
pink	126	19.1	7.7	4.5	0.4	ND	♟♟
pinto	120	14.3	7.8	7	0.7	Low	♟♟♟
refried beans, canned	119	12.9	6.9	6.7	1.6	ND	♟♟♟
roman	121	12.8	8.3	8.9	0.4	ND	♟♟♟
white	125	16.8	8.7	5.7	0.3	Low	♟♟♟
winged	127	12.9	9.2	ND	5	ND	♟♟♟
yardlong	101	14.8	7.1	3.3	0.4	ND	♟♟♟
yellow	128	13.2	8.1	9.2	1	ND	♟♟♟
Peanuts							
dry-roasted w/salt, 1 oz	166	3.8	6.7	2.3	14.1	Low	♟♟
oil-roasted w/salt, 1/4 cup	216	2.1	10.1	3.4	18.9	Low	♟
peanuts, raw, 1/4 cup	207	2.8	9.4	3.1	18	Low	♟
peanut butter, chunky, 2 tbsp	188	4.7	8	2.1	15.9	ND	♟♟♟
peanut butter, reduced sodium, 2 tbsp	203	4.9	7.7	2.1	16	ND	♟♟♟
peanut butter, smooth, 2 tbsp	192	4	8	1.9	16.7	ND	♟♟♟

ND = No Data

Food	Cal	Net Carb	Protein	Fiber	Total Fat	Glycemic Load	Advice
Peas, 1/2 cup							
cowpeas (blackeyes), cooked	100	12.3	6.7	5.6	0.5	Low	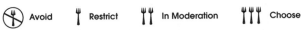
green peas, cooked, 1 cup	134	16.2	8.6	8.8	0.4	Low	
split, cooked	116	12.6	8.2	8.2	0.4	Low	
Soy Products							
bacon, Yves, 1 strip	25	1	3	0	1	ND	
beans, cooked, 1/2 cup	149	3.4	14.3	5.2	7.7	Low	
burger, Boca original vegan, 1 burger	70	2	13	4	1	ND	
Canadian bacon, Yves, 3 slices	80	1	17	1	0.5	ND	
cheese							
soy cheese, 1 oz	60	6	3	0	2	ND	
sandwich slices, Soya Kaas, 1 slice	40	0	4	ND	3	ND	
sandwich slices, Soyco, 1 slice	60	1	6	0	3	ND	
cream cheese, Soya Kaas Natural Cream Cheese Alternative, plain, 2 tbsp	80	0	3	ND	9	ND	
cream cheese, Tofutti Better than Cream Cheese, plain, 2 tbsp	120	13	1	0	7	ND	
creamer, Silk, plain, 1 tbsp	15	1	0	0	1	ND	
lunchmeat, deli slices (*see also* Processed Meats)							
bologna, Smart Deli, 4 slices	60	2	15	2	0	ND	

 Avoid   Restrict   In Moderation   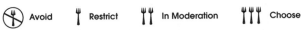 Choose

Food	Cal	Net Carb	Protein	Fiber	Total Fat	Glycemic Load	Advice
ham, Smart Deli, 4 slices	90	4	16	1	0	ND	🍴🍴
original, Tofurkey, 3 slices	150	15	16	2	2	ND	🍴🍴
pastrami, Smart Deli, 4 slices	60	1	13	0	0	ND	🍴🍴
pepperoni, Smart Deli, 13 slices	45	2	8	1	0	ND	🍴🍴
turkey, Smart Deli, 4 slices	80	3	15	1	0	ND	🍴🍴
meat, ground, Yves, 1/3 cup	60	2	10	3	0.5	ND	🍴🍴🍴
meatballs, Yves, 5 balls	110	4	16	3	2.5	ND	🍴🍴🍴
miso, 1/4 cup	142	15.5	8.1	3.7	4.2	ND	🍴🍴🍴
nuggets, breaded w/whole wheat, 4 nuggets	120	13	13	2	2	ND	🚫🍴
sausage (*see also* Processed Meats)							
soy sausage links, Yves, 2 links	70	1	11	2	2	ND	🍴🍴🍴
soy sausage patties, Yves, 2 patties	80	2	11	2	2	ND	🍴🍴🍴
soy sausage, Italian, Tofurkey, 3.5 oz	270	4	29	8	13	ND	🍴🍴🍴
soy meal, defatted, raw, 1 cup	414	49	54.8	ND	2.9	ND	🚫🍴
soymilk, Silk, 1 cup (240ml) (*see also* Dairy and Eggs)							
chai	140	19	6	0	4	Low	🍴
chocolate	140	21	5	2	3.5	Low	🍴
plain	100	7	7	1	4	Low	🍴🍴🍴
unsweetened	90	3	7	1	4	Low	🍴🍴🍴

Food	Cal	Net Carb	Protein	Fiber	Total Fat	Glycemic Load	Advice
vanilla	100	9	6	1	3.5	Low	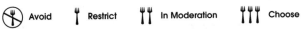
tempeh, Lightlife, 4 oz	210	4	19	10	9	ND	
tofu, 1/5 block							
firm, 365 Organic	90	1	11	ND	5	ND	
firm, White Wave	110	2	11	2	6	ND	
silken	45	2	4	0	2.5	ND	
soft	60	0	6	1	3	ND	
yogurt, soy (*see also* Dairy and Eggs)							
Silk, 6 oz	60	28	4	1	2	Med.	
Stonyfield O'Soy, 6 oz	170	29	7	4	2	Med.	
Whole Soy, 6 oz	150	26	5	1	2.5	Med.	

 Avoid   Restrict    In Moderation   Choose

Meat

ANIMAL PRODUCTS HAVE GOTTEN A BAD RAP OVER THE LAST FEW decades because of their fat content, but it's time to set the record straight. Saturated fat is not the demon it's been made out to be, and you shouldn't judge whether a food is "good" or "bad" based on the saturated fat content.

The problem with animal products stems from the way the animals are raised. Many factory-farmed animals are treated with a chemical soup of antibiotics, steroids, growth hormones, and other nasty things that don't belong in their bodies, let alone ours. They're fed grains—not their natural diet of grass—so their fat content is much higher in inflammatory omega-6s than in the healthier omega-3s. And because they don't get much exercise, they're not very lean.

As far as I'm concerned, it's way more important to consider where your meat comes from than to worry about its fat content. Though more expensive and not always practical, try to buy only grass-fed beef raised using organic farming standards. There are five foods I strongly recommend you buy organic: milk, eggs, strawberries, coffee (if at all), and meat.

Some of the ratings have more to do with the sheer caloric value of the meat than anything else. After all, just because something is low in carbohydrates does not mean it's a free food. In general, meats that were less than 200 calories or so got a "Choose" rating, assuming everything else looked okay. That doesn't mean you can never eat the higher-calorie cuts, just that you should always be aware of your low-carb caloric budget.

Remember—calories aren't the whole story, but they still count for something!

MEAT

Food	Cal	Net Carb	Protein	Fiber	Total Fat	Advice
Beef, 3 oz serving unless noted						
breakfast strips, 3 slices	153	0.5	10.6	0	11.7	ψψψ
brisket, braised, trimmed to 1/8" fat unless noted						
corned beef, brisket	213	0	15.4	0	16.1	ψψ
flat half, lean w/fat	246	0	24.5	0	15.7	ψψ
flat half, lean only, trimmed to 0" fat	174	0	28.3	0	5.9	ψψψ
flat half, lean only	167	0	28.2	0	5.1	ψψψ
point half, lean w/fat, trimmed to 0" fat	304	0	20	0	24.2	ψ
point half, lean w/fat	297	0	20.7	0	23.1	ψψ
point half, lean only, trimmed to 0" fat	207	0	23.8	0	11.7	ψψψ
whole, lean w/fat, trimmed to 0" fat	247	0	22.8	0	16.6	ψψ
whole, lean w/fat	281	0	22	0	20.8	ψψ
whole, lean only, trimmed to 0" fat	185	0	25.3	0	8.6	ψψψ
chuck, trimmed to 1/8" fat unless noted						
arm pot roast, lean w/fat, braised	257	0	25.6	0	16.3	ψψ
arm pot roast, lean only, braised, trimmed to 0" fat	178	0	28.1	0	6.5	ψψψ
blade roast, lean w/fat, braised	290	0	22.8	0	21.4	ψψ
blade roast, lean only, braised, trimmed to 0" fat	215	0	26.4	0	11.3	ψψ

 Avoid   Restrict   In Moderation   Choose

Food	Cal	Net Carb	Protein	Fiber	Total Fat	Advice
clod roast, lean w/fat, roasted, trimmed to 0" fat	176	0	21.8	0	9.2	ŸŸŸ
clod roast, lean only, roasted, trimmed to 0" fat	146	0	22.8	0	5.4	ŸŸŸ
clod steak, lean w/fat, braised, trimmed to 0" fat	187	0	24.5	0	9.2	ŸŸŸ
clod steak, lean only, braised, trimmed to 0" fat	163	0	25.4	0	6.1	ŸŸŸ
mock tender steak, lean w/fat, broiled, trimmed to 0" fat	136	0	22	0	4.7	ŸŸŸ
mock tender steak, lean only, broiled, trimmed to 0" fat	136	0	22	0	4.6	ŸŸŸ
top blade, lean w/fat, broiled, trimmed to 0" fat	184	0	21.9	0	10	ŸŸŸ
top blade, lean only, broiled, trimmed to 0" fat	173	0	22.2	0	8.6	ŸŸŸ
flank						
lean w/fat, broiled, trimmed to 0" fat	160	0	23.5	0	7	ŸŸŸ
lean only, broiled, trimmed to 0" fat	158	0	23.7	0	6.3	ŸŸŸ
ground beef (80% lean meat/20% fat)						
crumbles, pan-browned	231	0	23	0	14.8	ŸŸ
loaf, baked	216	0	21.5	0	13.7	ŸŸ
patty, broiled	230	0	21.9	0	15.2	ŸŸ
patty, pan-broiled	209	0	20.4	0	13.6	ŸŸŸ
ground beef (95% lean meat/5% fat)						
crumbles, pan-browned	164	0	24.8	0	6.4	ŸŸŸ
loaf, baked	148	0	23.2	0	5.4	ŸŸŸ

ND = No Data

Food	Cal	Net Carb	Protein	Fiber	Total Fat	Advice
patty, broiled	145	0	22.4	0	5.6	
patty, pan-broiled	139	0	21.9	0	5.1	
patties, frozen, broiled, medium	240	0	20.8	0	16.7	
liver, braised	162	4.4	24.7	0	4.5	
frankfurters (*see* **Processed Meats**)						
bottom round, trimmed to 0" fat						
lean w/fat, braised	181	0	26.5	0	7.5	
lean w/fat, roasted	159	0	23.3	0	6.6	
lean only, braised	173	0	26.9	0	6.5	
lean only, roasted	150	0	23.6	0	5.5	
eye of round, trimmed to 0" fat						
lean w/fat, roasted	145	0	24.5	0	4.6	
lean only, roasted	141	0	24.6	0	4	
full cut round						
lean w/fat, broiled, trimmed to 1/8" fat	200	0	23.4	0	11	
porterhouse steak, trimmed to 0" fat						
lean w/fat, broiled	235	0	20.4	0	16.4	
lean only, broiled	180	0	22.2	0	9.5	
ribs, small end rib eye (ribs 10–12)						
lean w/fat, broiled, trimmed to 0" fat	210	0	23.2	0	12.5	

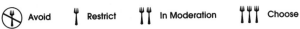 Avoid   Restrict   In Moderation   Choose

Food	Cal	Net Carb	Protein	Fiber	Total Fat	Advice
lean only, broiled, trimmed to 0" fat	164	0	25	0	6.4	⑂⑂⑂
ribs, large end (ribs 6–9)						
lean w/fat, roasted, trimmed to 0" fat	300	0	19.7	0	24	⑂⑂
lean only, roasted, trimmed to 0" fat	202	0	23.4	0	11.4	⑂⑂⑂
ribs, shortribs						
lean w/fat, braised	400	0	18.3	0	35.7	⊘
lean only, braised	251	0	26.2	0	15.4	⑂⑂
ribs, small end (ribs 10–12)						
lean w/fat, broiled, trimmed to 0" fat	252	0	21.2	0	17.9	⑂⑂
lean w/fat, roasted, trimmed to 1/8" fat	290	0	19.2	0	23.1	⑂⑂
lean only, broiled, trimmed to 0" fat	181	0	23.8	0	8.8	⑂⑂⑂
lean only, broiled, trimmed to 1/8" fat	172	0	24.1	0	7.7	⑂⑂⑂
ribs, whole (ribs 6–12), lean w/fat, roasted, trimmed to 1/8" fat	298	0	19.4	0	23.9	⑂⑂
skirt steak, trimmed to 0" fat						
inside skirt steak, lean w/fat, broiled	187	0	22.2	0	10.2	⑂⑂⑂
inside skirt steak, lean only, broiled	174	0	22.7	0	8.6	⑂⑂⑂
outside skirt steak, lean w/fat, broiled	217	0	20	0	14.6	⑂⑂
outside skirt steak, lean only, broiled	198	0	20.6	0	12.2	⑂⑂⑂
sirloin, bottom, trimmed to 0" fat						
butt, tri-tip roast, lean w/fat, roasted	184	0	23.7	0	9.2	⑂⑂⑂

Food	Cal	Net Carb	Protein	Fiber	Total Fat	Advice
butt, tri-tip roast, lean only, roasted	177	0	24	0	8.2	ŸŸŸ
butt, tri-tip steak, lean w/fat, broiled	225	0	25.5	0	12.9	ŸŸ
butt, tri-tip steak, lean only, broiled	212	0	26.1	0	11.2	ŸŸ
tri-tip roast, lean w/fat, roasted	177	0	22.1	0	9.4	ŸŸŸ
tri-tip, lean only, roasted	155	0	22.7	0	7.1	ŸŸŸ
sirloin, top, trimmed to 0" fat						
lean w/fat, broiled	183	0	25	0	8.5	ŸŸŸ
lean only, broiled	162	0	25.8	0	5.8	ŸŸŸ
T-bone steak, trimmed to 0" fat						
lean w/fat, broiled	210	0	20.6	0	13.5	ŸŸ
lean only, broiled	161	0	22.1	0	7.4	ŸŸŸ
tenderloin, trimmed to 0" fat						
lean w/fat, broiled	200	0	23.1	0	11.2	ŸŸŸ
lean only, broiled	175	0	24	0	8.1	ŸŸŸ
tip round, trimmed to 0" fat						
lean w/fat, roasted	162	0	23.9	0	6.7	ŸŸŸ
lean only, roasted	150	0	24.4	0	5	ŸŸŸ
top loin, trimmed to 0" fat						
lean w/fat, broiled	180	0	23.9	0	8.7	ŸŸŸ
lean only, broiled	168	0	24.3	0	7.1	ŸŸŸ

 Avoid Restrict In Moderation Choose
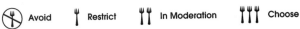

Food	Cal	Net Carb	Protein	Fiber	Total Fat	Advice
top round, trimmed to 0" fat						
lean w/fat, braised	178	0	30.3	0	5.4	♈♈♈
lean w/fat, broiled	158	0	26.9	0	5	♈♈♈
lean only, braised	169	0	30.7	0	4.3	♈♈♈
lean only, broiled	158	0	27	0	4.8	♈♈♈
Bison, 3 oz serving						
top sirloin, lean only, 1" steak, broiled	145	0	23.8	0	4.8	♈♈♈
chuck, shoulder clod, lean only, 3-5 lb roast, braised	164	0	28.7	0	4.6	♈♈♈
ground, pan-broiled	202	0	20.2	0	12.9	♈♈♈
lean only, roasted	122	0	24.2	0	2.1	♈♈♈
Lamb, 3 oz serving						
cubed for stew or kabob, lean only, braised, trimmed to 1/4" fat	190	0	28.6	0	7.5	♈♈♈
cubed for stew or kabob, lean only, broiled, trimmed to 1/4" fat	158	0	23.9	0	6.2	♈♈♈
foreshank, lean w/fat, braised, trimmed to 1/8" fat	207	0	24.1	0	11.4	♈♈♈
ground lamb, broiled	241	0	21	0	16.7	♈♈
leg, trimmed to 1/8" fat						
shank half, lean w/fat, choice, roasted	184	0	22.7	0	9.7	♈♈♈
sirloin half, lean w/fat, choice, roasted	241	0	21.2	0	16.7	♈♈
whole, lean w/fat, choice, roasted	206	0	22.3	0	12.3	♈♈

Food	Cal	Net Carb	Protein	Fiber	Total Fat	Advice
loin, trimmed to 1/8" fat						
lean w/fat, choice, broiled	252	0	22.2	0	17.5	
lean w/fat, choice, roasted	246	0	19.8	0	18	
rib, trimmed to 1/8" fat						
lean w/fat, choice, broiled	289	0	19.6	0	22.8	
lean w/fat, choice, roasted	290	0	18.6	0	23.4	
shoulder, trimmed to 1/8" fat						
arm, lean w/fat, choice, braised	286	0	26.4	0	19.3	
arm, lean w/fat, choice, roasted	227	0	19.5	0	15.9	
arm, lean w/fat, broiled	229	0	21.2	0	15.3	
blade, lean w/fat, choice, braised	288	0	24.6	0	20.3	
blade, lean w/fat, choice, broiled	227	0	20	0	15.7	
blade, lean w/fat, choice, roasted	230	0	19.2	0	16.3	
whole, lean w/fat, choice, braised	287	0	25	0	20	
whole, lean w/fat, choice, broiled	228	0	20.3	0	15.6	
whole, lean w/fat, choice, roasted	229	0	19.3	0	16.2	
Pork, Cured						
breakfast strips, 3 slices	156	0.4	9.8	0	12.5	
bacon, 1 slice						
Canadian-style, grilled	43	0.3	5.7	0	2	

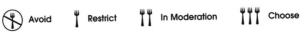

Avoid   Restrict   In Moderation   Choose

Food	Cal	Net Carb	Protein	Fiber	Total Fat	Advice
broiled, pan-fried, or roasted	43	0.1	3	0	3.3	ŸŸŸ
microwaved	37	0.1	2.9	0	2.8	ŸŸŸ
ham, 3 oz unless noted						
boneless, extra lean and regular, roasted	140	0.4	18.7	0	6.5	ŸŸŸ
canned, extra lean and regular, roasted	142	0.4	17.8	0	7.2	ŸŸ
canned, regular (approximately 13% fat), roasted	192	0.4	17.5	0	12.9	ŸŸ
low-sodium, lean w/fat	146	0.3	19	0	7.1	ŸŸŸ
patties, grilled, 1 patty	205	1	8	0	18.5	ŸŸŸ
whole, lean w/fat, roasted	207	0	18.3	0	14.3	ŸŸŸ
whole, lean only, roasted	133	0	21.3	0	4.7	ŸŸŸ
shoulder, 3 oz serving						
arm picnic, lean w/fat, roasted	238	0	17.4	0	18.2	ŸŸ
arm picnic, lean only, roasted	144	0	21.2	0	6	ŸŸŸ
blade roll, lean w/fat, roasted	244	0.3	14.7	0	20	ŸŸ
Pork, Fresh 3 oz serving						
backribs, lean w/fat, roasted	314	0	20.6	0	25.1	Ÿ
ground	252	0	21.8	0	17.7	ŸŸ
leg (ham)						
rump half, lean w/fat, roasted	214	0	24.6	0	12.1	ŸŸ

Food	Cal	Net Carb	Protein	Fiber	Total Fat	Advice
rump half, lean only, roasted	175	0	26.3	0	6.9	♈♈♈
shank half, lean w/fat, roasted	246	0	21.5	0	17.1	♈♈
shank half, lean only, roasted	183	0	24	0	8.9	♈♈♈
whole, lean w/fat, roasted	232	0	22.8	0	15	♈♈
whole, lean only, roasted	179	0	25	0	8	♈♈♈
loin chops, blade						
lean w/fat, braised	275	0	18.6	0	21.6	♈♈
lean w/fat, broiled	272	0	19.1	0	21.1	♈♈
lean only, braised	191	0	21.3	0	11.1	♈♈♈
lean only, broiled	199	0	21.6	0	11.8	♈♈♈
loin chops, center loin						
lean w/fat, braised	210	0	23.8	0	12	♈♈♈
lean w/fat, broiled	204	0	24.4	0	11.1	♈♈♈
lean only, braised	172	0	25.3	0	7.1	♈♈♈
lean only, broiled	172	0	25.7	0	6.9	♈♈♈
loin chops, center rib						
lean w/fat, braised	217	0	22.4	0	13.4	♈♈
lean w/fat, broiled	221	0	23.5	0	13.4	♈♈
lean only, braised	179	0	23.8	0	8.6	♈♈♈

 Avoid    Restrict   In Moderation   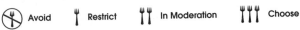 Choose

Food	Cal	Net Carb	Protein	Fiber	Total Fat	Advice
lean only, broiled	184	0	25	0	8.5	♈♈♈
loin roasts						
bone-in, lean w/fat, roasted	275	0	20.2	0	20.9	♈♈
bone-in, lean only, roasted	210	0	22.6	0	12.6	♈♈♈
center loin, bone-in, lean w/fat, roasted	199	0	22.4	0	11.4	♈♈♈
center loin, bone-in, lean only, roasted	169	0	23.4	0	7.7	♈♈♈
center rib, boneless, lean w/fat, roasted	214	0	22.9	0	12.9	♈♈
center rib, boneless, lean only, roasted	182	0	24.5	0	8.6	♈♈♈
ribs						
country-style, lean w/fat, roasted	279	0	19.9	0	21.5	♈♈
country-style, lean only, roasted	210	0	22.6	0	12.6	♈♈♈
spareribs, lean w/fat, braised	337	0	24.7	0	25.8	♈
shoulder						
arm picnic, lean w/fat, roasted	269	0	20	0	20.4	♈♈
arm picnic, lean only, roasted	194	0	22.7	0	10.7	♈♈♈
blade, Boston (roasts), lean w/fat, roasted	229	0	19.6	0	16	♈♈
blade, Boston (roasts), lean only, roasted	197	0	20.6	0	12.2	♈♈♈
blade, Boston (steaks), lean w/fat, braised	271	0	24.4	0	18.5	♈♈
blade, Boston (steaks), lean w/fat, broiled	220	0	21.7	0	14.1	♈♈
blade, Boston (steaks), lean only, braised	232	0	26.4	0	13.2	♈♈

Food	Cal	Net Carb	Protein	Fiber	Total Fat	Advice
blade, Boston (steaks), lean only, broiled	193	0	22.7	0	10.7	↑↑↑
whole, lean w/fat, roasted	248	0	19.8	0	18.2	↑↑
whole, lean only, roasted	196	0	21.5	0	11.5	↑↑↑
sirloin chops						
lean w/fat, braised	161	0	22.6	0	7.1	↑↑
lean w/fat, broiled	177	0	25.9	0	7.3	↑↑
lean only, braised	149	0	23	0	5.6	↑↑
lean only, broiled	164	0	26.5	0	5.7	↑↑
sirloin roasts						
boneless, lean w/fat, roasted	176	0	24.2	0	8	↑↑↑
boneless, lean only, roasted	168	0	24.5	0	7	↑↑↑
tenderloin						
lean w/fat, broiled	171	0	25.4	0	6.9	↑↑↑
lean w/fat, roasted	147	0	23.6	0	5.1	↑↑↑
lean only, broiled	159	0	25.9	0	5.4	↑↑↑
lean only, roasted	139	0	23.9	0	4.1	↑↑↑
top loin chops						
lean w/fat, braised	160	0	24.1	0	6.3	↑↑↑
lean w/fat, broiled	154	0	25	0	5.2	↑↑↑

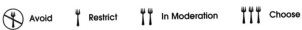 Avoid   Restrict   In Moderation   Choose

Food	Cal	Net Carb	Protein	Fiber	Total Fat	Advice
lean w/fat, pan-fried	218	0	24.7	0	12.6	♟♟
lean only, braised	145	0	24.5	0	4.5	♟♟♟
lean only, broiled	141	0	25.4	0	3.6	♟♟♟
lean only, pan-fried	191	0	25.9	0	8.9	♟♟♟
top loin roasts						
boneless, lean w/fat, roasted	192	0	24.5	0	9.7	♟♟♟
lean only, roasted	165	0	25.7	0	6.1	♟♟♟
whole loin						
lean w/fat, braised	203	0	23.2	0	11.6	♟♟♟
lean w/fat, broiled	206	0	23.2	0	11.8	♟♟♟
lean w/fat, roasted	211	0	23	0	12.5	♟♟♟
lean only, braised	173	0	24.3	0	7.8	♟♟♟
lean only, broiled	178	0	24.3	0	8.3	♟♟♟
lean only, roasted	178	0	24.3	0	8.2	♟♟♟
Veal, 3 oz serving						
breast						
whole, boneless, lean w/fat, braised	226	0	22.9	0	14.3	♟♟
whole, boneless, lean only, braised	185	0	25.8	0	8.3	♟♟♟
cubed for stew, lean only, braised	160	0	29.7	0	3.7	♟♟♟
ground, broiled	146	0	20.7	0	6.4	♟♟♟

Food	Cal	Net Carb	Protein	Fiber	Total Fat	Advice
leg (top round)						
lean w/fat, braised	179	0	30.7	0	5.4	♈♈♈
lean w/fat, roasted	136	0	23.6	0	4	♈♈♈
lean only, braised	173	0	31.2	0	4.3	♈♈♈
lean only, roasted	128	0	23.9	0	2.9	♈♈♈
loin						
lean w/fat, braised	241	0	25.7	0	14.6	♈♈
lean w/fat, roasted	184	0	21.1	0	10.5	♈♈♈
lean only, braised	192	0	28.5	0	7.8	♈♈♈
lean only, roasted	149	0	22.4	0	5.9	♈♈♈
rib						
lean w/fat, braised	213	0	27.6	0	10.7	♈♈
lean w/fat, roasted	194	0	20.4	0	11.9	♈♈♈
lean only, braised	185	0	29.3	0	6.6	♈♈♈
lean only, roasted	150	0	21.9	0	6.3	♈♈♈
shank (fore and hind)						
lean w/fat, braised	162	0	26.8	0	5.3	♈♈♈
lean only, braised	150	0	27.4	0	3.7	♈♈♈
shoulder, arm						
lean w/fat, braised	201	0	28.6	0	8.7	♈♈♈

 Avoid   Restrict   In Moderation   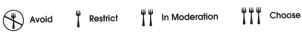 Choose

Food	Cal	Net Carb	Protein	Fiber	Total Fat	Advice
lean w/fat, roasted	156	0	21.6	0	7	🍴🍴🍴
lean only, braised	171	0	30.4	0	4.5	🍴🍴🍴
lean only, roasted	139	0	22.2	0	4.9	🍴🍴🍴
sirloin						
lean w/fat, braised	214	0	26.6	0	11.2	🍴🍴
lean w/fat, roasted	172	0	21.4	0	8.9	🍴🍴🍴
lean only, braised	173	0	28.9	0	5.5	🍴🍴🍴
lean only, roasted	143	0	22.4	0	5.3	🍴🍴🍴

Nuts and Seeds

NUTS ARE SOME OF THE MOST PERFECT FOODS ON THE PLANET. Most are low in carbs and high in minerals, contain healthy fats, and typically have respectable amounts of fiber for a snack food. They got a bad rap during the days of the low-fat movement, but they're making a comeback and it's fully deserved. Nuts belong on your menu.

Like everything else, it's a question of how much and how often. While there are almost no "bad" nuts I can think of, those roasted in oil received lower ratings because they're usually roasted in cheap, processed oils that are heavy in omega-6 fats. Dry-roasted nuts almost always got a "Choose" rating. And pumpkin seeds were taken down a notch because they're so high in calories—try to choose the lower-calorie selections when you can.

Cashews are below average because they're relatively high in carbs. Chinese chestnuts are up there too, but they're so low in calories (for a one-ounce portion) that they earned a high rating. Again, any of these nuts and seeds works well if you stay conscious of the portion size and the carb content.

Studies have shown significant health benefits—even weight-loss benefits—associated with consumption of nuts, but you have to be careful. It's not a great idea to buy those family-sized bags of almonds and nibble on them all day long. You'll want to keep your portions to ¼ cup or 1 ounce, depending on the nut. And if your weight loss seems stalled, nuts are frequently a culprit, possibly because they're so easy to overeat.

You can't go wrong with this terrific class of food if, as with everything else, you consume consciously!

NUTS AND SEEDS

Food	Cal	Net Carb	Protein	Fiber	Total Fat	Glycemic Load	Advice
Nuts							
acorns, raw, 1 oz	110	11.6	1.7	0	6.8	ND	🍴🍴🍴
almonds, 1/4 cup							
blanched	211	3.4	8	3.8	18.4	Low	🍴🍴🍴
dry-roasted	206	2.6	7.6	4.1	18.2	Low	🍴🍴🍴
honey-roasted	214	5.1	6.5	4.9	18	Low	🍴🍴
oil-roasted	238	2.8	8.3	4.1	21.7	Low	🍴
raw	207	2.9	7.6	4.2	18.1	Low	🍴🍴🍴
brazilnuts, 1/4 cup	230	1.7	5	2.6	23.3	Low	🍴🍴
cashews, dry-roasted, 1/4 cup	197	10.2	5.2	1	15.9	Low	🍴
cashews, oil-roasted, 1/4 cup	187	8.6	5.4	1.1	15.4	Low	🍴
cashews, raw, 1/4 cup	180	6	5	2	14	Low	🍴🍴🍴
chestnuts, Chinese, cooked, 1 oz	43	9.5	0.8	ND	0.2	ND	🍴🍴🍴
chestnuts, European, cooked, 1 oz	37	7.9	0.6	ND	0.4	ND	🍴🍴🍴
chestnuts, Japanese, cooked, 1 oz	16	3.6	0.2	ND	0.1	ND	🍴🍴🍴
hazelnuts (filberts), dry-roasted, 1 oz	183	2.3	4.3	2.7	17.7	Low	🍴🍴🍴
hazelnuts (filberts), raw, 1/4 cup	210	2	4	3	21	Low	🍴🍴🍴
macadamia nuts, dry-roasted, 1/4 cup	240	1.6	2.6	2.7	25.5	Low	🍴🍴🍴

ND = No Data

Food	Cal	Net Carb	Protein	Fiber	Total Fat	Glycemic Load	Advice
macadamia nuts, raw, 1/4 cup	200	2	2	2	21	Low	ŤŤŤ
peanuts (*see* Legumes)							
pecans, dry-roasted, 1 oz	201	1.1	2.7	2.7	21.1	Low	ŤŤŤ
pecans, oil-roasted, 1 oz	203	1	2.6	2.7	21.3	Low	Ť
pine nuts, dry, 1/4 cup	227	3.2	4.6	1.3	23.1	ND	ŤŤŤ
pistachio nuts, dry-roasted, 1/4 cup	175	5	6.6	3.2	14.1	ND	ŤŤŤ
soynuts (*see* Legumes)							
walnuts, black, 1/4 cup, chopped	193	1	7.5	2.1	18.4	Low	ŤŤŤ
walnuts, English, 1/4 cup, halved	164	1.7	3.8	1.7	16.3	Low	ŤŤŤ
Nut and Seed Butters							
almond butter, 2 tbsp	203	5.6	4.8	1.2	18.9	ND	ŤŤŤ
cashew butter, 2 tbsp	188	8.2	5.6	0.6	15.8	ND	ŤŤŤ
Peanut Butter (*see* Legumes)							
sunflower seed butter, 1 tbsp	185	8.8	6.3	ND	15.3	ND	ŤŤŤ
tahini (sesame butter), 1 tbsp	89	1.8	2.6	1.4	8.1	ND	ŤŤŤ
Seeds							
cottonseed kernels, roasted, 1 tbsp	51	1.6	3.3	0.6	3.6	ND	ŤŤŤ
flaxseeds, 3 tbsp	140	5	5	6	10	ND	ŤŤŤ
pumpkin seed kernels, dried, 1/4 cup	187	4.8	8.5	1.3	15.8	ND	ŤŤŤ

 Avoid   Restrict   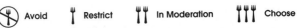 In Moderation   Choose

Food	Cal	Net Carb	Protein	Fiber	Total Fat	Glycemic Load	Advice
pumpkin seed kernels, roasted, 1/4 cup	296	5.4	18.7	2.2	23.9	ND	ꭹ
pumpkin seeds, whole, roasted, 1/4 cup	71	8.6	3	ND	3.1	ND	ꭹꭹꭹ
safflower seed kernels, dried, 1 oz	147	9.7	4.6	ND	10.9	ND	ꭹ
sesame seed kernels, dried, 1 tbsp	47	0.2	1.6	1	4.4	ND	ꭹꭹꭹ
sesame seed kernels, toasted, 1 tbsp	45	0.7	1.4	1.4	3.8	ND	ꭹꭹꭹ
sesame seeds, whole, dried, 1 tbsp	52	1	1.6	1.1	4.5	ND	ꭹꭹꭹ
sesame seeds, whole, roasted, 1 oz	160	3.3	4.8	4	13.6	ND	ꭹꭹꭹ
sunflower seed kernels, dried, 1/4 cup	205	3	8.2	3.8	17.9	ND	ꭹꭹꭹ
sunflower seed kernels, dry-roasted, 1/4 cup	186	4.1	6.2	3.6	15.9	ND	ꭹꭹꭹ
sunflower seed kernels, oil-roasted, 1/4 cup	208	2.7	7.2	2.3	19.4	ND	ꭹ
watermelon seed kernels, dried, 1/4 cup	150	4.1	7.7	ND	12.8	ND	ꭹꭹꭹ

Poultry

IN THE CASE OF POULTRY, THERE'S GOOD NEWS AND THERE'S bad news.

The good news: poultry is a great source of protein. And, contrary to popular belief, at least half the fat in poultry is monounsaturated. The calorie content is low and the carbs are nonexistent. What's not to like?

The bad news: poultry can be just as contaminated as red meat. Once again, the conditions under which the animals are raised determine how good for you the food will be. Horrendous factory-farming conditions produce birds that are far less healthy than their free-range, organically raised counterparts. Factory-farmed and processed birds are more likely to be loaded with antibiotics, hormones, and other nasty compounds. Instead of eating their natural foods, like worms and insects, they're fed grains and corn that are very likely sprayed with a cornucopia of potential toxins—and this starch- and carb-heavy diet has an enormous impact on the birds' fat content.

The bottom line: poultry is a wonderful food group, but you should always try to get organically raised, free-range chicken, turkey, and eggs. It may not make much of a difference in terms of carbs or weight loss, but it definitely makes a heck of a difference to your overall health.

POULTRY						
Food	Cal	Net Carb	Protein	Fiber	Total Fat	Advice
Chicken						
dark and light meat, broilers or fryers						
dark meat w/skin, fried, batter	253	0	18.6	0	15.8	🚫🍴
dark meat w/skin, fried, flour	242	3.5	23.1	0	14.4	🚫🍴
dark meat w/skin, roasted	215	0	22.1	0	13.4	🍴🍴🍴
dark meat w/skin, stewed	198	0	20	0	12.5	🍴🍴🍴
dark meat only, fried	203	2.2	24.6	0	9.9	🚫🍴
dark meat only, roasted	174	0	23.3	0	8.3	🍴🍴🍴
dark meat only, stewed	163	0	22.1	0	7.6	🍴🍴🍴
light meat w/skin, fried, batter	235	8.1	20	0	13.1	🚫🍴
light meat w/skin, fried, flour	209	1.5	25.9	0.1	10.3	🚫🍴
light meat w/skin, roasted	189	0	24.7	0	9.2	🍴🍴🍴
light meat w/skin, stewed	171	0	22.2	0	8.5	🍴🍴🍴
light meat only, fried	163	0.4	27.9	0	4.7	🚫🍴
light meat only, roasted	147	0	26.3	0	3.8	🍴🍴🍴
light meat only, stewed	135	0	24.6	0	3.4	🍴🍴🍴
breast, broilers or fryers						
w/skin, fried, batter	221	7.3	21.1	0.3	11.2	🚫🍴

Food	Cal	Net Carb	Protein	Fiber	Total Fat	Advice
w/skin, fried, flour	189	1.3	27.1	0.1	7.5	
w/skin, roasted	167	0	25.3	0	6.6	
w/skin, stewed	156	0	23.3	0	6.3	
meat only, fried	159	0.4	28.4	0	4	
meat only, roasted	140	0	26.4	0	3	
meat only, stewed	128	0	24.6	0	2.6	
drumstick, broilers or fryers						
w/skin, fried, batter	228	6.7	18.7	0.3	13.4	
w/skin, fried, flour	208	1.3	22.9	0.1	11.7	
w/skin, roasted	184	0	23	0	9.5	
w/skin, stewed	173	0	21.5	0	9	
meat only, fried	166	0	24.3	0	6.9	
meat only, roasted	146	0	24.1	0	4.8	
meat only, stewed	144	0	23.4	0	4.9	
leg, broilers or fryers						
w/skin, fried, batter	232	7.1	18.5	0.3	13.7	
w/skin, fried, flour	216	2	22.8	0.1	12.3	
w/skin, roasted	197	0	22.1	0	11.4	

 Avoid Restrict 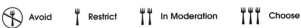 In Moderation Choose

Food	Cal	Net Carb	Protein	Fiber	Total Fat	Advice
w/skin, stewed	187	0	20.5	0	11	♙♙♙
meat only, fried	177	0.6	24.1	0	7.9	⊗
meat only, roasted	162	0	23	0	7.2	♙♙♙
meat only, stewed	157	0	22.3	0	6.9	♙♙♙
thigh						
w/skin, fried, batter	235	7.4	18.4	0.3	14.1	⊗
w/skin, fried, flour	223	2.6	22.7	0.1	12.7	⊗
w/skin, roasted	210	0	21.3	0	13.2	♙♙♙
w/skin, stewed	197	0	19.8	0	12.5	♙♙♙
meat only, fried	185	1	24	0	8.8	⊗
meat only, roasted	178	0	22.1	0	9.3	♙♙♙
meat only, stewed	166	0	21.3	0	8.3	♙♙♙
wing						
w/skin, fried, batter	275	9	16.9	0.3	18.5	⊗
w/skin, fried, flour	273	1.9	22.2	0.1	18.8	⊗
w/skin, roasted	246	0	22.8	0	16.5	♙♙♙
w/skin, stewed	212	0	19.4	0	14.3	♙♙♙
meat only, fried	179	0	25.6	0	7.8	⊗
meat only, roasted	173	0	25.9	0	6.9	♙♙♙

Food	Cal	Net Carb	Protein	Fiber	Total Fat	Advice
meat only, stewed	154	0	23.1	0	6.1	Choose
organ meat						
giblets, fried	235	3.7	27.7	0	11.4	Avoid
giblets, simmered	134	0.4	23.1	0	3.8	Choose
gizzard, all classes, simmered	124	0	25.8	0	2.3	Choose
liver, all classes, pan-fried	146	0.9	21.9	0	5.5	Choose
liver, all classes, simmered	142	0.7	20.8	0	5.5	Choose
canned chicken						
meat only, w/broth	140	0	18.5	0	6.8	Choose
no broth	156	0.7	21.5	0	6.9	Choose
capons						
giblets, simmered	139	0.7	22.4	0	4.6	Choose
w/skin and giblets and neck, roasted	192	0	24.1	0	9.9	Choose
w/skin, roasted	195	0	24.6	0	9.9	Choose
Cornish game hens						
w/skin, roasted	221	0	18.9	0	15.5	Choose
meat only, roasted	114	0	19.8	0	3.3	Choose
roasting chickens						
dark meat, meat only, roasted	151	0	19.8	0	7.4	Choose

 Avoid   Restrict   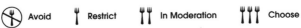 In Moderation   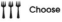 Choose

Food	Cal	Net Carb	Protein	Fiber	Total Fat	Advice
giblets, simmered	140	0.7	22.8	0	4.4	♟♟♟
light meat, meat only, roasted	130	0	23.1	0	3.5	♟♟♟
meat, w/skin, roasted	190	0	20.4	0	11.4	♟♟♟
meat only, roasted	142	0	21.3	0	5.6	♟♟♟
stewing chickens						
dark meat, meat only	219	0	23.9	0	13	♟♟♟
giblets, simmered	165	0.1	21.9	0	7.9	♟♟♟
light meat, meat only	181	0	28.1	0	6.8	♟♟♟
meat, w/skin	242	0	22.9	0	16	♟♟♟
meat only	201	0	25.9	0	10.1	♟♟♟
Duck, 3 oz serving						
meat, w/skin, roasted	286	0	16.1	0	24.1	♟♟
meat only, roasted	171	0	20	0	9.5	♟♟♟
young duckling, White Pekin, breast, w/skin, roasted	172	0	20.8	0	9.2	♟♟♟
young duckling, White Pekin, breast, meat only, broiled	119	0	23.5	0	2.1	♟♟♟
young duckling, White Pekin, leg, w/skin, roasted	184	0	22.7	0	9.7	♟♟♟
young duckling, White Pekin, leg, meat only, braised	151	0	24.7	0	5.1	♟♟♟
Goose, Pheasant, and Quail, 3 oz serving						
goose, domesticated, meat and skin, roasted	259	0	21.4	0	18.6	♟♟

Food	Cal	Net Carb	Protein	Fiber	Total Fat	Advice
goose, domesticated, meat only, roasted	202	0	24.6	0	10.8	🍴🍴🍴
pheasant, total edible	210	0	27.5	0	10.3	🍴🍴🍴
quail, total edible	199	0	21.3	0	12	🍴🍴🍴
Turkey, 3 oz serving unless noted						
all classes						
w/skin, roasted	161	0	24.4	0	6.3	🍴🍴🍴
dark meat, meat only, roasted	159	0	24.3	0	6.1	🍴🍴🍴
dark meat, w/skin, roasted	188	0	23.4	0	9.8	🍴🍴🍴
gizzard, simmered	105	0.3	18.5	0	3.3	🍴🍴🍴
leg, w/skin, roasted	177	0	23.7	0	8.4	🍴🍴🍴
light meat, meat only, roasted	133	0	25.4	0	2.7	🍴🍴🍴
light meat, w/skin, roasted	167	0	24.3	0	7.1	🍴🍴🍴
liver, simmered	232	1	17	0	17.5	🍴🍴🍴
wing, w/skin, roasted	195	0	23.3	0	10.6	🍴🍴🍴
bacon, 1 oz	107	0.9	8.3	0	7.8	🍴🍴🍴
canned, meat only, w/broth	139	0	20.1	0	5.8	🍴🍴🍴
fryer-roasters						
breast, w/skin, roasted	130	0	24.7	0	2.7	🍴🍴🍴

  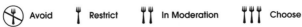

Avoid   Restrict   In Moderation   Choose

Food	Cal	Net Carb	Protein	Fiber	Total Fat	Advice
breast, meat only, roasted	115	0	25.6	0	0.6	♟♟♟
dark meat, w/skin, roasted	155	0	23.5	0	6	♟♟♟
dark meat, meat only, roasted	138	0	24.5	0	3.7	♟♟♟
leg, w/skin, roasted	144	0	24.2	0	4.6	♟♟♟
leg, meat only, roasted	135	0	24.8	0	3.2	♟♟♟
light meat, w/skin, roasted	139	0	24.5	0	3.9	♟♟♟
light meat, meat only, roasted	119	0	25.7	0	1	♟♟♟
wing, w/skin, roasted	176	0	23.5	0	8.4	♟♟♟
wing, meat only, roasted	139	0	26.2	0	2.9	♟♟♟
ground turkey	200	0	23.3	0	11.2	♟♟♟
patties, breaded, battered, fried	241	12.9	11.9	0.4	15.3	⊘
roast, boneless, light and dark meat, roasted	132	2.6	18.1	0	4.9	♟♟♟
smoked, bone removed						
drumstick w/skin	177	0	23.7	0	8.3	♟♟♟
light or dark meat w/skin	144	0	24.9	0	4.3	♟♟♟
light or dark meat w/skin	177	0	23.9	0	8.2	♟♟♟
wing w/skin	195	0	23.3	0	10.6	♟♟♟
young hen						
back, w/skin, roasted	216	0	22.5	0	13.3	♟♟♟

Food	Cal	Net Carb	Protein	Fiber	Total Fat	Advice
breast, w/skin, roasted	165	0	24.5	0	6.7	♗♗♗
dark meat, w/skin, roasted	197	0	23.3	0	10.9	♗♗♗
dark meat, meat only, roasted	163	0	24.2	0	6.6	♗♗♗
leg, w/skin, roasted	181	0	23.6	0	8.9	♗♗♗
light meat, w/skin, roasted	176	0	24.3	0	8	♗♗♗
light meat, meat only, roasted	137	0	25.4	0	3.2	♗♗♗
wing, w/skin, roasted	202	0	23.2	0	11.4	♗♗♗
young tom						
back, w/skin, roasted	202	0	22.8	0	11.6	♗♗♗
breast, w/skin, roasted	161	0	24.3	0	6.3	♗♗♗
dark meat, w/skin, roasted	184	0	23.4	0	9.2	♗♗♗
dark meat, meat only, roasted	157	0	24.4	0	5.9	♗♗♗
leg, w/skin, roasted	175	0	23.7	0	8.2	♗♗♗
light meat, w/skin, roasted	162	0	24.2	0	6.5	♗♗♗
light meat, meat only, roasted	131	0	25.4	0	2.5	♗♗♗
wing, w/skin, roasted	188	0	23.3	0	9.8	♗♗♗

 Avoid   Restrict   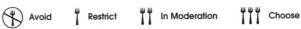 In Moderation   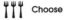 Choose

Prepared Foods

PREPARED FOODS ARE NOT MY FAVORITE CHOICE FOR A HEALTHY meal, but there are those times when opening a can or popping a TV dinner in the microwave seems like the only option. Try to make those times as infrequent as possible.

In this category, it really pays to read labels. Even when carbohydrate and calorie counts are low, sodium is usually very high and there are more unpronounceable chemicals than you can shake a stick at (and that includes many of the entrees with "healthy" on the labels!). Stick with the plain stuff—meat, vegetables, and soups. The health food section of your grocery will often have pretty interesting soup and chili selections, including some organic meals made with a minimum of chemicals. Try these. They're usually the best of the lot.

PREPARED FOODS

Food	Cal	Net Carb	Protein	Fiber	Total Fat	Advice
Boxed Entrees, 1 serving						
cheeseburger macaroni, Hamburger Helper	178	28.9	5	ND	4.7	
macaroni and cheese dinner, Kraft	259	46	11.3	1.5	2.6	
Canned Entrees, 1 serving						
beefaroni, macaroni w/beef in tomato sauce, Chef Boyardee	184	28.1	8.3	3	3	
beef ravioli in tomato and meat sauce, Chef Boyardee	229	33.2	8.4	3.7	5.4	
beef ravioli (mini) in tomato and meat sauce, Chef Boyardee	239	37.3	8.8	3.3	4.7	
chili w/beans, Hormel	240	25.3	16.6	8.4	4.4	
chili w/beans, Nestlè, Chef-Mate	412	17.9	17.7	11.1	25	
chili w/beans, Old El Paso	249	11.9	17.6	9.8	10.3	
chili, no beans, Hormel	175	13.4	15.3	2.8	5.9	
chili, no beans, Nestlè, Chef-Mate	430	14.6	18.6	3	31.6	
corned beef hash, Hormel	349	17.5	18.6	2.3	21.8	
corned beef hash, Nestlè, Chef-Mate	486	23	24.2	6.1	30.3	
roast beef hash, Hormel	385	19.4	21.3	3.5	23.7	
spaghetti and meatballs in tomato sauce, Chef Boyardee	250	31.9	9.1	2.2	8.6	

 Avoid   Restrict   In Moderation   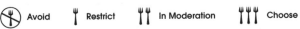 Choose

Food	Cal	Net Carb	Protein	Fiber	Total Fat	Advice
turkey chili w/beans, Hormel	175	16.6	16.2	5.5	2.4	🍴🍴🍴
vegetarian chili w/beans, Hormel	205	28.1	11.9	9.9	0.7	🚫
Frozen Entrees						
burgers and frankfurters						
burger crumbles, meatless, Morningstar Farms, 1 serving	116	0.8	11.1	2.5	6.5	🍴🍴🍴
Better'n Burgers, frozen, 1 patty	91	3.3	13.9	4.2	0.5	🍴🍴🍴
breakfast patties, meatless, 1 patty	79	1.7	9.9	2	2.8	🍴🍴🍴
deli franks, meatless, 1 serving	112	1	10.4	2.7	6.2	🍴🍴
garden veggie patties, Natural Touch, 1 patty	119	6.2	11.2	4	3.8	🍴🍴
spicy black bean burger, meatless, 1 patty	115	10.4	11.8	4.8	0.8	🍴🍴
vegan burgers, Natural Touch, 1 patty	91	3.3	13.9	4.2	0.5	🍴🍴
meat dinners, 1 serving						
bacon, egg, and cheese, Lean Pockets	150	19	7	2	4.5	🍴🍴
beef and bean burrito, Las Campanas	296	37.4	8.7	0.8	12.1	🚫
beef and cheddar stuffed sandwich, Hot Pockets	403	39.2	16.3	ND	20.2	🚫
beef macaroni, Healthy Choice	211	28.9	14.1	4.6	2.2	🚫
beef pot roast, Stouffer's Lean Cuisine	207	18.8	17.3	3.6	5.4	🍴🍴
beef sirloin Salisbury steak, Budget Gourmet Light and Healthy	261	26.7	18.4	7.2	5.9	🚫
beef stir-fry kit, Tyson	433	70.8	25.8	ND	5	🚫

ND = No Data

Food	Cal	Net Carb	Protein	Fiber	Total Fat	Advice
beef stroganoff and noodles, Marie Callender's	600	54.3	30.4	4.4	27	
cheeseburger, Lean Pockets	280	39	12	3	7	
creamed chipped beef, Stouffer's	175	7.1	9.9	ND	11.9	
ham and cheddar, Lean Pockets	280	37	14	3	7	
ham and cheese pocket, Red Baron Premium	356	36.2	14.9	ND	16.9	
ham 'n cheese stuffed sandwich, Hot Pockets	340	38.4	14.9	ND	14.2	
Italian sausage lasagna, Budget Gourmet	456	36.9	20.6	3	23.8	
lasagna w/meat and sauce, Stouffer's	277	23.3	18.7	3.2	10.8	
macaroni and beef in tomato sauce, Stouffer's Lean Cuisine	249	33.1	13.9	3.4	5.4	
macaroni and beef in tomato sauce, Weight Watchers	282	38	15.6	6.7	4.6	
meatballs and mozzarella, Lean Pockets	290	41	13	3	7	
meat loaf dinner, Banquet Extra Helping	612	27.3	29.1	6.3	40.1	
meat loaf w/tomato sauce, Healthy Choice	316	56.3	15.3	6.1	5	
mesquite beef w/barbecue sauce, Healthy Choice	320	33.3	21.4	5	9	
oriental beef w/vegetables and rice, Stouffer's Lean Cuisine	242	36.2	13.5	ND	4.8	
pepperoni pizza, Lean Pockets	280	39	14	3	7	
philly steak and cheese, Lean Pockets	280	37	13	3	7	

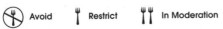

Avoid   Restrict   In Moderation   Choose

Food	Cal	Net Carb	Protein	Fiber	Total Fat	Advice
Salisbury steak in gravy, Stouffer's Homestyle	386	26.4	22.6	ND	21.2	🍴
Salisbury steak dinner, Banquet Extra Helping	782	40.1	27.1	7	54.2	🚫🍴
Salisbury steak meal, Banquet	398	24.2	15.3	3.5	25	🍴
Salisbury steak w/mushroom gravy, Healthy Choice	326	41.8	18	6.2	6.9	🚫🍴
sliced beef meal, Banquet	270	14.7	26.4	4.1	10.1	🍴🍴
spaghetti w/meatballs, low-fat, Michelina's	312	42.4	13.6	6.2	7.1	🚫🍴
spaghetti w/meatballs and sauce, Stouffer's Lean Cuisine	299	34.9	18	4.6	7.5	🚫🍴
stuffed peppers w/beef, Stouffer's Lean Cuisine	189	15.6	7.9	5.3	8.1	🍴🍴
Swedish meatballs w/pasta, Stouffer's Lean Cuisine	276	28.6	21.7	2.6	7.2	🚫🍴
veal parmigiana meal w/tomato sauce, Banquet	362	28.2	12.6	6.6	19.1	🚫🍴
poultry dinners, 1 serving						
barbecue glazed chicken and sauce w/mixed vegetables, Weight Watchers	217	25.9	18.8	ND	4.4	🍴
cacciatore chicken, Healthy Choice	266	30.9	22	5	4	🚫🍴
chicken, broccoli, and cheddar pocket sandwich, Weight Watchers On-the-Go	266	39.6	13.4	ND	6.1	🚫🍴
chicken, broccoli, and cheddar stuffed croissant, Hot Pockets	301	37.5	11.4	1.4	11	🚫🍴
chicken, cheddar, and broccoli, Lean Pockets	260	36	11	3	7	🚫🍴
chicken and vegetables w/vermicelli, Stouffer's Lean Cuisine	252	27.1	18.7	5	5.6	🚫🍴

Food	Cal	Net Carb	Protein	Fiber	Total Fat	Advice
chicken enchilada and Mexican-style rice, Stouffer's	376	43.9	12.5	4.5	14.8	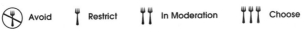
chicken enchilada suiza, Stouffer's Lean Cuisine	298	47.7	11.5	4.3	4.8	
chicken enchilada suiza, Weight Watchers	283	29.6	16.1	3.6	9.7	
chicken enchilada suprema in green chili sauce, Healthy Choice	298	41.8	13	4.2	6.8	
chicken fajita, Lean Pockets	260	35	11	3	7	
chicken fajita kit, Tyson	129	17.4	8	ND	3.3	
chicken mesquite w/barbecue sauce, Tyson	321	40.7	17.8	4.3	7.8	
chicken parmesan, Lean Pockets	280	40	13	3	7	
chicken pie, Stouffer's	572	33.4	23.2	3.1	37.1	
chicken pot pie, Marie Callender's	501	44.2	12.4	ND	30.6	
chicken pot pie, Banquet	382	35	9.9	1	22	
chicken teriyaki, Healthy Choice	268	34.3	17.1	2.8	5.6	
Cosmic Chicken Nuggets, w/macaroni in cheese sauce, Kid Cuisine	524	49.8	17.7	3.1	26.7	
country roast turkey, Healthy Choice	223	24.7	19	3.1	3.9	
escalloped noodles and chicken, Marie Callender's	292	28.3	9.6	ND	15.6	
French recipe chicken, Budget Gourmet Light	178	3.1	23	6.1	5.6	

 Avoid   Restrict   In Moderation   Choose

Food	Cal	Net Carb	Protein	Fiber	Total Fat	Advice
fried chicken meal, Banquet	470	33	21.5	2.1	27	⊘
Lunch Express chicken alfredo, Stouffer's Lean Cuisine	373	28.8	19	3.8	18.5	⊘
Lunch Express rice and chicken stir-fry, Stouffer's Lean Cuisine	270	33.6	11.7	5.9	7.4	⊘
mesquite chicken BBQ, Healthy Choice	310	42.1	18.1	6	5	⊘
roasted chicken w/garlic sauce, Tyson	214	17.9	16.9	3.6	6.7	♈♈
roast turkey medallions and mushrooms, Weight Watchers Smart Ones	214	31.5	15.1	3.1	1.7	⊘
teriyaki chicken breast, Budget Gourmet Light and Healthy	317	48.3	18.7	4	3.9	⊘
turkey and gravy w/dressing meal, Banquet	280	31.1	14	2.9	9.9	⊘
turkey w/gravy, Marie Callender's	504	51.9	31.1	ND	19	⊘
vegetable dinners, 1 serving						
broccoli in cheese-flavored sauce, Green Giant, 1 cup	113	15	3.9	ND	4.2	♈♈♈
cheddar broccoli potatoes, Healthy Choice	328	47	13	6	7	⊘
spinach au gratin, Budget Gourmet	222	9.2	6.7	2.3	16.6	♈♈♈
Pizzas, frozen, 1 serving						
deluxe w/sausage, peppers, and mushrooms, Celeste	386	33.2	16.7	ND	20.7	⊘
deep dish sausage, Tony's D'Primo	391	40.6	12.4	ND	19.9	⊘
deluxe French bread w/sausage, pepperoni, and mushroom, Stouffer's	429	41	16.1	3.5	20.7	⊘

Food	Cal	Net Carb	Protein	Fiber	Total Fat	Advice
Italian-style pastry crust w/sausage, pepperoni, mushrooms, peppers, onions, Tony's Supreme	400	39.1	15.8	ND	20	
Party Pizza, crisp crust combination, Totino's	385	36	14.1	ND	20.4	
pepperoni w/Italian-style pastry crust, Tony's	406	36.3	14.9	ND	22.4	
pepperoni and sausage, Tombstone	317	25.6	13.3	1.7	17.2	
pepperoni, Red Baron	442	36	18	ND	25.1	
Pizza Rolls, pepperoni, Totino's	385	37.2	14.4	2.3	18.9	
premium deep dish singles, pepperoni, Red Baron	480	47.9	16	ND	25	
sausage and mushroom, Tombstone	306	31.2	14.4	ND	13.7	
supreme, sausage, mushrooms, and pepperoni, Red Baron	344	31.8	13.6	ND	18.1	

Soup, 1 cup unless noted

bean

Food	Cal	Net Carb	Protein	Fiber	Total Fat	Advice
black bean, canned, prepared w/water	116	15.4	5.6	4.4	1.5	
w/ham, chunky, ready-to-serve	231	15.9	12.6	11.2	8.5	
w/pork, canned, prepared w/water	172	14.2	7.9	8.6	6	

beef

Food	Cal	Net Carb	Protein	Fiber	Total Fat	Advice
beef bouillon, canned, ready-to-serve	17	0.1	2.7	0	0.5	
beef bouillon, powder, prepared w/water	20	1.9	1.3	0	0.7	

 Avoid   Restrict   In Moderation   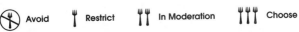 Choose

Food	Cal	Net Carb	Protein	Fiber	Total Fat	Advice
beef mushroom, canned, prepared w/water	73	6.1	5.8	0.2	3	♟♟♟
beef noodle, canned, prepared w/water	83	8.3	4.8	0.7	3.1	♟♟♟
beef noodle, dehydrated, prepared w/water	40	5.2	2.2	0.8	0.8	♟♟♟
beef stroganoff, chunky, ready-to-serve, 1 serving	235	20.2	12.2	1.4	11	♟
chili beef, canned, prepared w/water	170	12	6.7	9.5	6.6	♟♟♟
chunky, ready-to-serve	170	18.2	11.7	1.4	5.1	♟♟♟
vegetable beef, dehydrated, prepared w/water	53	7.5	2.9	0.5	1.1	♟♟♟
vegetable beef, ready-to-serve, 1 serving	128	5.2	18.1	4.4	2	♟♟♟
cheese, canned, prepared w/milk	231	15.2	9.5	1	14.6	♟
cheese, canned, prepared w/water	156	9.5	5.4	1	10.5	♟♟
chicken						
broth, canned, prepared w/water	38	0.9	4.9	0	1.4	♟♟♟
broth, cubes, prepared w/water	22	1.4	1.3	0	1.1	♟♟♟
chicken w/dumplings, canned, prepared w/water	96	5.6	5.6	0.5	5.5	♟♟♟
chicken corn chowder, chunky, ready-to-serve, 1 serving	238	15.8	7.4	2.2	15.1	♟
chicken mushroom, canned, prepared w/water	132	9.1	4.4	0.2	9.2	♟♟♟
chunky, ready-to-serve	170	15.1	12.1	1.4	6.3	♟♟♟
gumbo, canned, prepared w/water	56	6.4	2.6	2	1.4	♟♟♟
chicken rice, canned, prepared w/water	60	6.5	3.5	0.7	1.9	♟♟♟

Food	Cal	Net Carb	Protein	Fiber	Total Fat	Advice
chicken noodle						
w/celery and carrots, homestyle, ready-to-serve, 1 serving	95	9.5	6.4	ND	3.4	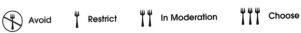
canned, prepared w/water	75	8.7	4.1	0.7	2.5	
dehydrated, prepared w/water	55	8.6	2	0.2	1.3	
chicken vegetable						
canned, prepared w/water	75	7.6	3.6	1	2.8	
dehydrated, prepared w/water	50	7.8	2.7	ND	0.8	
clam chowder						
Manhattan-style, canned, prepared w/water	78	10.7	2.2	1.5	2.2	
Manhattan-style, chunky, ready-to-serve	134	15.9	7.3	2.9	3.4	
New England–style, canned, prepared w/milk	164	15.1	9.5	1.5	6.6	
New England–style, canned, prepared w/water	95	10.9	4.8	1.5	2.9	
crab, ready-to-serve	76	9.6	5.5	0.7	1.5	
cream-based						
asparagus, canned, prepared w/water	85	10.2	2.3	0.5	4.1	
celery, canned, prepared w/water	90	8.1	1.7	0.7	5.6	
chicken, canned, prepared w/water	117	9.1	3.4	0.2	7.4	
mushroom, canned, prepared w/water	129	8.8	2.3	0.5	9	
mushroom, ready-to-serve	129	10.6	2.4	0.5	9	

 Avoid   Restrict In Moderation Choose

Food	Cal	Net Carb	Protein	Fiber	Total Fat	Advice
onion, canned, prepared w/water	107	11.7	2.8	1	5.3	♈♈♈
potato, canned, prepared w/water	73	11	1.8	0.5	2.4	♈♈♈
shrimp, canned, prepared w/water	90	8	2.8	0.2	5.2	♈♈♈
escarole, ready-to-serve	27	1.8	1.5	ND	1.8	♈♈♈
fish stock	40	0	5.3	0	1.9	♈♈♈
gazpacho, ready-to-serve	46	3.9	7.1	0.5	0.2	♈♈♈
green pea, canned, prepared w/water	165	23.7	8.6	2.8	2.9	⊘
lentil w/ham, ready-to-serve	139	20.2	9.3	ND	2.8	♈♈♈
lentil, vegetarian, canned, Walnut Acres, ready-to-serve	130	18	7	8	0	♈♈♈
minestrone, canned, prepared w/water	82	10.2	4.3	1	2.5	♈♈♈
minestrone, chunky, ready-to-serve	127	14.9	5.1	5.8	2.8	♈♈♈
mushroom barley, canned, prepared w/water	73	11	1.9	0.7	2.3	♈♈♈
mushroom w/beef stock, canned, prepared w/water	85	8.6	3.2	0.7	4	♈♈♈
onion, canned, prepared w/water	58	7.2	3.8	1	1.7	♈♈♈
onion, dehydrated, prepared w/water	27	4.1	1.1	1	0.6	♈♈♈
oyster stew, canned, prepared w/milk	135	9.8	6.2	0	7.9	♈♈♈
oyster stew, canned, prepared w/water	58	4.1	2.1	ND	3.8	♈♈♈
potato ham chowder, chunky, ready-to-serve, 1 serving	192	12	6.5	1.4	12.5	♈♈♈

Food	Cal	Net Carb	Protein	Fiber	Total Fat	Advice
ramen noodles, dehydrated, 1 serving, dry	190	26.5	3.9	1	7.2	
split pea w/ham, canned, prepared w/water	190	25.7	10.3	2.3	4.4	
split pea w/ham, chunky, ready-to-serve	185	22.7	11.1	4.1	4	
tomato, canned, prepared w/milk	161	19.6	6.1	2.7	6	⅃
tomato, canned, prepared w/water	85	16.1	2.1	0.5	1.9	⅃⅃⅃
tomato rice, canned, prepared w/water	119	20.4	2.1	1.5	2.7	
turkey noodle, canned, prepared w/water	68	7.9	3.9	0.7	2	⅃⅃⅃
turkey vegetable, canned, prepared w/water	72	8.1	3.1	0.5	3	⅃⅃⅃
turkey, chunky, ready-to-serve	135	14.1	10.2	ND	4.4	⅃⅃⅃
vegetable						
chunky, ready-to-serve	122	17.8	3.5	1.2	3.7	⅃⅃⅃
vegetarian, canned, prepared w/water	72	11.5	2.1	0.5	1.9	⅃⅃⅃

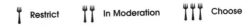 Avoid    Restrict   ⅃⅃ In Moderation   ⅃⅃⅃ Choose

Processed Meats

OKAY, LET ME BE HONEST. I'VE NEVER MET A PROCESSED MEAT I LIKED. My own opinion is that half the reason meat-eating diets got such a bad rap in the first place is because the populations studied were consuming hot dogs and bologna as their prime sources of meat, not to mention maintaining a diet devoid of fiber and vegetables. If the groups tested had been eating healthy, free-range, grass-fed animal products, complemented with a ton of vegetables, fiber, and good fats, meat-eating would never have received bad press in the first place.

In this category, the foods that worry me most are hot dogs, anything smoked (because of carcinogens), "lunch meats" of mysterious origin, and of course, the original processed "meat food," Spam. I've given some processed lunch meats, such as salami, a "Restrict" rating because I know people love them, and from a blood-sugar point of view they're fine. I just can't bring myself to recommend that you eat them often. If these meats aren't your main source of protein, I suppose it's okay.

The processed meats category does contain some acceptable foods. The good guys are foods like deli turkey, which, if you're lucky, is pretty fresh and pure. Some companies are conscientious about sliced turkey and their products can be recommended without reservation. Even sausage—if you know what's in it—can be acceptable. Be sure the processed meats you choose are nitrate-free. It won't make a difference in terms of weight loss, but it will to your general health, and I actually care about that just as much as I do your weight.

PROCESSED MEATS

Food	Cal	Net Carb	Protein	Fiber	Total Fat	Advice
Canned Meat, 1 oz serving						
corned beef, cured	71	0	7.7	0	4.2	
ham, chopped	68	0.1	4.6	0	5.3	
pork and chicken, minced, includes SPAM Lite	58	0.5	4.6	0	4.1	
pork w/ham, minced, includes SPAM	94	0.5	3.8	0	8.4	
Frankfurters, 1 frank						
beef	188	2.3	6.4	0	16.9	
beef, low fat	133	0.9	6.8	0	11.1	
beef and pork	174	0	6.6	1.4	15.8	
beef and pork, low-fat	88	2.5	6.3	0	5.7	
beef, pork, and turkey, fat-free	46	3.4	7.7	0	0	
chicken	116	3.1	5.8	0	8.8	
meatless	163	2.7	13.7	2.7	9.6	
soy dogs, Yves, 1 dog	50	0	11	1	0	
turkey	102	0.7	6.4	0	8	

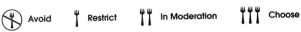

Avoid   Restrict   In Moderation   Choose

Food	Cal	Net Carb	Protein	Fiber	Total Fat	Advice
Lunch meat						
beef and pork, 1 oz serving						
beef, thin sliced	50	1.6	8	0	1.1	⅋⅋
chopped beef, cured, smoked	37	0.5	5.7	0	1.2	⊘
corned beef, Carl Buddig, cooked, chopped	40	0.3	5.5	0	1.9	⅋⅋
liverwurst, pork	92	0.6	4	0	8.1	⊘
liverwurst spread	86	1	3.5	0.7	7.2	⊘
pastrami, cured	98	0.9	4.8	0	8.2	⅋
pastrami, 98% fat-free	27	0.4	5.6	0	0.3	⅋
salami (Genoa), Oscar Mayer	110	0.3	5.9	0	9.4	⅋
salami (hard), Oscar Mayer	104	0.5	7.3	0	8.1	⅋
bologna, 1 oz serving						
beef	87	1.1	2.9	0	7.9	⅋
beef, low-fat	64	0.9	3.6	0	5.3	⅋
beef and pork	86	1.6	4.3	0	7	⅋
beef and pork, low-fat	64	0.7	3.2	0	5.4	⅋
Lebanon bologna	52	0.1	5.4	0	3	⅋
chicken, 1 oz serving						
breast, Louis Rich, oven-roasted deluxe	28	0.7	5.1	0	0.6	⅋⅋⅋
breast, Oscar Mayer, oven-roasted, fat-free	24	0.5	5.2	0	0.2	⅋⅋⅋

ND = No Data

Food	Cal	Net Carb	Protein	Fiber	Total Fat	Advice
oven-roasted, fat-free, sliced	22	0.6	4.6	0	0.1	🍴🍴🍴
ham, 1 oz serving						
boiled, Oscar Mayer	29	0.3	4.7	0	1.1	🍴🍴🍴
minced	75	0.5	4.6	0	5.9	🍴🍴
sliced, extra lean (approximately 5% fat)	37	0.3	5.4	0	1.4	🍴🍴🍴
sliced, regular (approximately 11% fat)	46	0.7	4.7	0.4	2.4	🍴🍴🍴
smoked, Oscar Mayer	28	0	4.7	0	1	🚫
96% fat-free, baked, Oscar Mayer	29	0.5	4.6	0	1	🍴🍴🍴
lunch meat, other						
barbecue loaf, pork, beef	49	1.8	4.5	0	2.3	🍴
beef, loaved	86	0.8	4	0	7.3	🍴
luncheon loaf (spiced), Oscar Mayer	66	2	3.8	0	4.7	🍴
Old-Fashioned Loaf, Oscar Mayer	65	2.2	3.7	0	4.6	🍴
Olive Loaf, chicken, pork, turkey, Oscar Mayer	74	1.9	2.8	0	6.1	🍴
sandwich spread, pork, chicken, beef, Oscar Mayer	67	4.3	1.8	0.1	4.7	🚫
soy lunchmeat, deli slices (*see also* Legumes)						
bologna, Smart Deli, 4 slices	60	2	15	2	0	🍴🍴
ham, Smart Deli, 4 slices	90	4	16	1	0	🍴🍴
original, Tofurkey, 3 slices	150	15	16	2	2	🍴🍴

 Avoid   Restrict   In Moderation   Choose

Food	Cal	Net Carb	Protein	Fiber	Total Fat	Advice
pastrami, Smart Deli, 4 slices	60	1	13	0	0	♟♟
pepperoni, Smart Deli, 13 slices	45	2	8	1	0	♟♟
turkey, Smart Deli, 4 slices	80	3	15	1	0	♟♟
turkey, 1 oz serving						
breast meat	29	1.1	4.8	0.1	0.5	♟♟♟
deli-cut, white, rotisserie	32	2.1	3.8	0.1	0.9	♟♟♟
turkey bologna	59	1.2	3.2	0.1	4.5	♟♟♟
turkey ham, cured turkey thigh meat	35	0.5	4.9	0.1	1.4	♟♟♟
turkey pastrami	40	0.5	5.2	0	1.8	♟♟♟
turkey salami	41	0.1	4.3	0	2.6	♟♟♟
Sausage, 1 oz unless noted						
beef sausage, fresh, cooked	94	0.1	5.2	0	7.9	♟
beef sausage, pre-cooked	115	0	4.4	0	10.7	♟
beef sausage, smoked	88	0.7	4	0	7.6	⊘
bratwurst, beef and pork, smoked, 3 oz	252	1.7	10.4	0	22.4	⊘
bratwurst, pork, cooked, 3 oz	281	2.1	11.7	0	24.8	⊘
chicken and beef sausage, smoked	84	0	5.2	0	6.8	⊘
Italian pork sausage, cooked, 3 oz	275	1.3	17	0	21.8	⊘
Italian sweet sausage, links, 3 oz	125	1.8	13.6	0	7.1	♟♟

Food	Cal	Net Carb	Protein	Fiber	Total Fat	Advice
Italian turkey sausage, smoked, 3 oz	134	3.2	12.8	0.8	7.4	
kielbasa, Polish, turkey and beef, smoked	64	1.1	3.7	0	5	
kielbasa, Tofurkey, meatless, 3.5 oz	240	4	26	8	12	ΥΥΥ
knockwurst, pork, beef	87	0.9	3.2	0	7.9	
link sausage, pork	110	0.6	6.3	0	9	Υ
pepperoni, pork, beef	130	0.7	5.7	0.4	11.3	
pepperoni, turkey, Hormel Pillow Pak Sliced	69	1.1	8.8	0	3.3	ΥΥΥ
Polish beef sausage w/chicken, hot	73	1	5	0	5.5	ΥΥ
Polish pork sausage, 1 oz	92	0.5	4	0	8.1	
pork, 1 link	204	0.1	9.7	0.1	18	
pork sausage, fresh, cooked	96	0	5.5	0	8	Υ
pork sausage, pre-cooked	107	0	4.1	0	9.9	Υ
salami, beef	73	0.5	3.6	0	6.3	Υ
salami, beef and pork	71	0.6	4	0	5.7	Υ
salami, turkey	42	0.1	4.3	0	2.6	ΥΥ
salami, dry or hard, pork	115	0.5	6.4	0	9.6	
salami, Italian, pork	119	0.3	6.1	0	10.4	

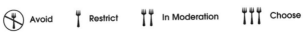

 Avoid   Υ Restrict   ΥΥ In Moderation   ΥΥΥ Choose

Food	Cal	Net Carb	Protein	Fiber	Total Fat	Advice
soy sausage links, Yves, 2 links	70	1	11	2	2	ŢŢŢ
soy sausage patties, Yves, 2 patties	80	2	11	2	2	ŢŢŢ
soy sausage, Italian, Tofurkey, 3.5 oz	270	4	29	8	13	ŢŢŢ
turkey and pork sausage, patty or link	86	0.2	6.4	0	6.4	ŢŢ
turkey sausage, fresh	54	0	6.8	0	3	ŢŢŢ
turkey sausage, reduced-fat, brown and serve	57	3	4.8	0.1	2.9	ŢŢŢ
Vienna sausage, beef and pork, 1 sausage	45	0.3	1.7	0	4	ŢŢ

Sauces, Condiments, and Seasonings

THERE ARE TWO WORDS TO LOOK FOR ON NUTRITION LABELS OF sauces, condiments, and seasonings: calories and chemicals. Some salad dressings—blue cheese, for example—may be fine from a carb point of view, but should be used sparingly on account of their high calorie content. Others are very low in calories, but contain loads of chemicals and artificial additives. At the risk of repeating myself for the millionth time, read the labels and consume consciously.

And as long as I'm repeating myself: pay attention to serving size. Notice that the recommended portion for salad dressing is two tablespoons. Don't super-size. Just because a dressing received a "Choose" rating in the Advice column doesn't mean you can serve it with a ladle! In fact, that's probably the number one mistake most people make with sauces, salad dressings, and the like. No one measures, everyone pours, and believe me, those calories (and carbs) really add up.

As far as seasonings go, the more the better. They've all received the highest rating. Many of these herbs have medicinal properties. Fenugreek and cinnamon both have beneficial effects on blood sugar. I tell my clients to use cinnamon as often as possible.

Even with high-sugar items, almost all of which received an "Avoid" rating, there are exceptions to the rule. A little cold-processed, organic honey (the cloudy kind, not the kind that comes in a bear) is fine once in a great while. I sometimes prepare myself a cleansing drink of hot water, lemon, cayenne pepper, and...maple syrup! If you do this, use grade-B syrup, which has far more nutrients than the other grades—but be sure to use it very sparingly and on special occasions.

SAUCES, CONDIMENTS, AND SEASONINGS

Food	Cal	Net Carb	Protein	Fiber	Total Fat	Advice
Condiments						
catsup, 1 tbsp	14	3.4	0.3	0.2	0.1	⊘
catsup, low-calorie, Carb Options, 1 tbsp	5	1	0	0	0	🍴🍴🍴
catsup, low-carb, Atkins Quick Quisine, 1 tbsp	10	1	0	1	0	🍴🍴🍴
hot pepper chili sauce, green, 1 tbsp	3	0.5	0.1	0.3	0	🍴🍴🍴
hot pepper chili sauce, red, 1 tbsp	3	0.5	0.1	0.1	0.1	🍴🍴🍴
hot sauce, 1 tsp	1	0.1	0	0	0	🍴🍴🍴
mustard, yellow, 1 tsp	3	0.2	0.2	0.2	0.2	🍴🍴🍴
relish, sweet pickle, 1 tbsp	20	5.1	0.1	0.2	0.1	🍴🍴
salsa, 1/2 cup	36	6	1.7	2.1	0.3	🍴🍴🍴
salsa, green jalapena, 2 tbsp	10	1.1	0.3	0.3	0.3	🍴🍴🍴
soy sauce, tamari, 1 tbsp	11	0.9	1.9	0.1	0	🍴🍴🍴
steak sauce, low-carb, Atkins Quick Quisine, 1 tbsp	5	1	0	0	0	🍴🍴🍴
sweeteners						
brown sugar, 1 tsp	17	4.5	0	0	0	⊘
granulated sugar, 1 packet	11	2.8	0	0	0	⊘
granulated sugar, 1 cube	9	2.3	0	0	0	⊘
honey, 1 tbsp	64	17.3	0.1	0	0	⊘

Food	Cal	Net Carb	Protein	Fiber	Total Fat	Advice
powdered sugar, 1 tsp	10	2.5	0	0	0	
sugar substitute, Equal, 1 packet	0	<1	0	0	0	restrict
sugar substitute, Splenda (sucralose)	0	<1	0	0	0	choose
tabasco sauce, 1 tsp	1	0	0.1	0	0	choose
taco sauce, green, 1 tbsp	4	0.8	0.1	0.1	0.1	choose
taco sauce, red, 1 tbsp	7	1.2	0.2	0.1	0.1	choose
teriyaki sauce, 1 tbsp	15	2.9	1.1	0	0	moderation
teriyaki sauce, low-carb, Atkins Quick Quisine, 1 tbsp	10	1	0	0	1	choose
tomato chili sauce, 1 tbsp	18	4.8	0.4	0.1	0.1	choose
vinegar, distilled, 1 tbsp	2	0.9	0	0	0	choose
vinegar, balsamic, 1 tbsp	5	1	0	ND	0	choose
Worcestershire sauce, 1 tbsp	11	3.3	0	0	0	choose

Preserves and Fruit Spreads, 1 tbsp

Food	Cal	Net Carb	Protein	Fiber	Total Fat	Advice
apple butter, all natural	20	4	0	1	0	restrict
apple butter, made w/sugar	30	8	0	0	0	
apple butter, Smucker's	45	11	0	0	0	
jam and preserves	56	13.6	0.1	0.2	0	
jams and preserves, made w/saccharin	18	7.2	0	0.3	0	restrict

 Avoid   Restrict   In Moderation   Choose

Food	Cal	Net Carb	Protein	Fiber	Total Fat	Advice
jam and jelly, Smucker's, all flavors	50	13	0	0	0	🚫🍴
low-sugar fruit spread, Fifty 50*	10	1	0	0	0	🍴🍴🍴
low-sugar preserves, Smucker's, all flavors	25	6	0	0	0	🍴🍴
no-sugar strawberry spread, Sorbee Zero Sugar*	15	1	0	ND	0	🍴🍴🍴
no-sugar orange marmalade, Sorbee Zero Sugar*	20	1	0	ND	0	🍴🍴🍴
Salad Dressings, 2 tbsp						
bacon and tomato	98	0.5	0.5	0.1	11	🍴🍴🍴
bacon vinaigrette, Maple Grove Farms, low-carb and sugar-free	90	1	0	ND	9	🍴🍴🍴
balsamic vinaigrette						
Annie's Naturals	100	3	0	ND	10	🍴🍴🍴
fat-free, Maple Grove Farms	5	1	0	ND	0	🍴🍴🍴
Seeds of Change	60	6	0	0	4	🍴🍴🍴
Wishbone	60	3	0	0	5	🍴🍴🍴
basil, Seeds of Change	60	6	0	0	4.5	🍴🍴🍴
blue cheese						
regular	151	2.2	1.4	0	16	🍴
fat-free	39	7.5	0.7	1.2	0.3	🍴🍴🍴
low-calorie	30	0.9	1.5	0	2.2	🍴🍴🍴

*contains sugar alcohols

Food	Cal	Net Carb	Protein	Fiber	Total Fat	Advice
reduced-calorie	28	4.2	0.7	0	0.9	♈♈♈
caesar	155	0.9	0.4	0	17	♈
caesar, low-calorie	33	5.6	0.1	0	1.3	♈♈♈
caesar, low-carb, Marzetti	120	1	1	0	13	♈♈
coleslaw dressing	125	7.6	0.3	0	11	♈
coleslaw dressing, reduced-fat	112	13.5	0	0.1	6.8	
Dijon vinaigrette, Seeds of Change	60	6	0	0	4	♈♈♈
French						
regular	146	5	0.3	0	14	
fat-free	42	9.6	0.1	0.7	0.1	♈♈
reduced-calorie	64	8.6	0.1	0	4.2	♈♈
reduced-fat	74	9	0.2	0.4	4.3	♈♈
honey Dijon, fat-free, Maple Grove Farms	40	9	0	1	0	♈
honey mustard, low-fat, Annie's Naturals	45	6	0	ND	2	♈♈
Italian						
regular	86	3.1	0.1	0	8.3	♈♈♈
creamy, Wishbone	110	4	1	0	10	♈♈
creamy, low-carb, Marzetti	160	1	1	0	17	♈

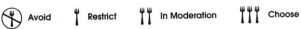

 Avoid   Restrict   In Moderation   Choose

Food	Cal	Net Carb	Protein	Fiber	Total Fat	Advice
fat-free	13	2.3	0.3	0.2	0.2	♟♟♟
reduced-calorie	56	1.8	0.1	0.1	5.6	♟♟♟
reduced-fat	22	1.4	0.1	0	1.9	♟♟♟
Tuscan, low-carb, Marzetti	110	1	0	0	12	♟♟
mayonnaise	100	0	0	0	11	♟♟
mayonnaise, low-calorie	32	2.2	0	0	2.7	♟♟♟
mayonnaise, made w/tofu	48	0.4	0.9	0.2	4.7	♟♟♟
Miracle Whip Free, nonfat	27	4.4	0.1	0.6	0.9	♟♟
Miracle Whip Light	74	4.6	0.2	0	6	♟♟
oil and vinegar	144	0.8	0	0	16	♟♟♟
olive oil vinaigrette, lite, Ken's	60	3	0	0	6	♟♟♟
peppercorn	151	0.9	0.3	0	17	♟
peppercorn ranch, fat-free, Ken's	30	6	1	1	0	♟♟♟
poppyseed, fat-free, Maple Grove Farms	50	11	1	0	0	♟♟♟
ranch						
regular	158	1.9	0.3	0.2	16	♟
fat-free	38	8.5	0.1	0	0.6	♟♟♟
low-carb, Marzetti	150	1	0	0	16	♟
reduced-fat	72	4.9	0.3	0.3	5.5	♟♟♟

Food	Cal	Net Carb	Protein	Fiber	Total Fat	Advice
raspberry vinaigrette, low-fat, Annie's Naturals	35	5	0	ND	1.5	ŤŤŤ
raspberry vinaigrette, fat-free, Maple Grove Farms	35	9	0	ND	0	ŤŤŤ
red wine vinaigrette, Wishbone	80	9	0	0	5	ŤŤŤ
Russian	148	3.1	0.5	0	15	Ť
Russian, low-calorie	45	8.7	0.2	0.1	1.3	ŤŤŤ
sesame ginger, Annie's Naturals	100	4	1	ND	9	ŤŤ
sesame seed	133	2.3	0.9	0.3	14	ŤŤ
sweet and sour	5	1.2	0	0	0	ŤŤŤ
Thousand Island	118	4.4	0.4	0.3	11	ŤŤ
Thousand Island, reduced-fat	61	6.3	0.3	0.4	3.9	ŤŤŤ
Thousand Island, fat-free	42	8.3	0.2	1.1	0.5	ŤŤŤ
Sauces and Gravies						
Alfredo sauce, dry mix, 2 tbsp	62	7.1	2.2	ND	2.7	Ť
barbecue sauce, 1/8 cup	23	3.6	0.6	0.4	0.6	Ť
barbecue sauce, low-carb, Atkins Quick Quisine, 1 tbsp	15	1	0	ND	1	ŤŤŤ
bearnaise sauce, dehydrated, 1/8 cup	8	1.3	0.3	ND	0.2	ŤŤ
cheese sauce, 1/8 cup	55	2	2.1	0.2	4.2	ŤŤ
curry sauce, dry, 1/4 cup	30	3.5	0.7	ND	1.6	ŤŤŤ

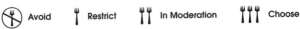 Avoid   Ť Restrict   ŤŤ In Moderation   ŤŤŤ Choose

Food	Cal	Net Carb	Protein	Fiber	Total Fat	Advice
enchilada sauce, 1/8 cup	10	1.2	0.1	0.2	0.4	🍴🍴🍴
fish sauce, 1 tbsp	6	0.7	0.9	0	0	🍴🍴🍴
gravy, 1/2 cup						
au jus, canned	19	3	1.4	0	0.2	🍴🍴🍴
beef, canned	62	5.1	4.4	0.5	2.8	🍴🍴🍴
chicken, canned	94	6	2.3	0.5	6.8	🍴🍴🍴
mushroom, canned	60	6	1.5	0.5	3.2	🍴🍴🍴
turkey, canned	61	5.6	3.1	0.5	2.5	🍴🍴🍴
hoisin sauce, 1 tbsp	35	6.7	0.5	0.4	0.5	🍴🍴
hollandaise sauce, w/butterfat, dehydrated, 1/8 cup	31	1.7	0.6	0.1	2.6	🍴🍴🍴
hollandaise sauce, w/vegetable oil, dehydrated, 1/8 cup	8	1.3	0.3	0	0.2	🍴🍴🍴
hollandaise sauce, w/butterfat, dehydrated, prepared w/water, 1/8 cup	30	1.6	0.6	0.1	2.5	🍴🍴🍴
hot dog chili sauce, Chef-Mate, 1/2 cup	69	7.5	2.7	1.7	2.4	🍴
lemon sauce, LJ Minor, 2 tbsp	43	10.2	0.1	0	0.2	🍴
marinara sauce, 1/2 cup	71	8.3	1.8	2	2.6	🍴🍴
mole poblano sauce, 1/2 cup	205	11	4.4	5.2	14	🚫
mushroom sauce, dehydrated, 1/8 cup	10	1.6	0.4	ND	0.3	🍴🍴🍴
nacho cheese sauce, Ortega, 1/4 cup	128	3.6	5.2	0.4	10	🍴🍴

Food	Cal	Net Carb	Protein	Fiber	Total Fat	Advice
oyster sauce, 1 tbsp	9	1.9	0.2	0.1	0	🍴🍴🍴
pasta sauce, meat flavor, Prego, 1/2 cup	140	18	2	3	5	🍴🍴
pasta sauce, Bella Vista, low-carb, 1/2 cup	70	4	2	2	5	🍴🍴🍴
plum sauce, 1 tbsp	35	8	0.2	0.1	0.2	🍴🍴🍴
soy sauce, tamari, 1 tbsp	11	0.9	1.9	0.1	0	🍴🍴🍴
steak sauce, low-carb, Atkins Quick Quisine, 1 tbsp	5	1	0	0	0	🍴🍴🍴
stir-fry sauce, LJ Minor, 1 tbsp	16	2.4	0.2	0	0.7	🍴🍴🍴
stroganoff sauce, dehydrated, 1/8 cup	25	3.9	0.9	0.1	0.7	🍴🍴🍴
sweet and sour sauce, dehydrated, 1/8 cup	37	8.9	0.1	0.2	0	🍴
tomato sauce						
herbs and cheese, 1/2 cup	72	9.8	2.6	2.7	2.4	🍴🍴
mushroom, 1/2 cup	43	8.5	1.8	1.8	0.2	🍴🍴
onion, 1/2 cup	51	10	1.9	2.2	0.2	🍴🍴
onion, green pepper, and celery, 1/2 cup	51	9.2	1.2	1.8	0.9	🍴🍴
regular, 1/2 cup	39	7.2	1.6	1.8	0.3	🍴🍴
Spanish-style, 1/2 cup	40	7.1	1.8	1.7	0.3	🍴🍴
white sauce						
dehydrated, 1/8 cup	12	1.2	0.3	0.1	0.7	🍴🍴🍴

 Avoid   Restrict   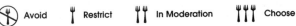 In Moderation   Choose

Food	Cal	Net Carb	Protein	Fiber	Total Fat	Advice
medium, 1/4 cup	92	5.6	2.4	0.1	6.6	♉♉
thick, 1/4 cup	116	7.1	2.5	0.2	8.6	♉♉
thin, 1/4 cup	66	4.5	2.4	0.1	4.2	♉♉
Seasonings, 1 tsp unless noted						
allspice, ground	5	1	0.1	0.4	0.2	♉♉♉
anise seed	7	0.8	0.4	0.3	0.3	♉♉♉
basil, dried, 1 tbsp	11	0.9	0.7	1.8	0.2	♉♉♉
basil, fresh, 1 tbsp	1	0	0.1	0.2	0	♉♉♉
bay leaf	2	0.3	0.1	0.2	0.1	♉♉♉
black pepper	5	0.8	0.2	0.6	0.1	♉♉♉
capers, canned, 1 tbsp, drained	2	0.1	0.2	0.3	0.1	♉♉♉
caraway seeds	7	0.3	0.4	0.8	0.3	♉♉♉
cardamom, ground	6	0.8	0.2	0.6	0.1	♉♉♉
cayenne pepper	6	0.5	0.2	0.5	0.3	♉♉♉
celery seed	8	0.6	0.4	0.2	0.5	♉♉♉
chervil, dried	1	0.2	0.1	0.1	0	♉♉♉
chili powder	8	0.5	0.3	0.9	0.4	♉♉♉
cider vinegar, 1 tbsp	2	0.9	0	0	0	♉♉♉
cinnamon, ground	6	0.6	0.1	1.2	0.1	♉♉♉

Food	Cal	Net Carb	Protein	Fiber	Total Fat	Advice
cloves, ground	7	0.6	0.1	0.7	0.4	♥♥♥
coriander leaf, dried	2	0.2	0.1	0.1	0	♥♥♥
coriander seed	5	0.2	0.2	0.8	0.3	♥♥♥
cumin seed	8	0.7	0.4	0.2	0.5	♥♥♥
curry powder	6	0.5	0.3	0.7	0.3	♥♥♥
dill seed	6	0.8	0.3	0.4	0.3	♥♥♥
dill weed, dried	3	0.5	0.2	0.1	0	♥♥♥
dill weed, fresh, 1/4 cup	1	0.2	0.1	0	0	♥♥♥
fennel seed	7	0.3	0.3	0.8	0.3	♥♥♥
fenugreek seed	12	1.3	0.9	0.9	0.2	♥♥♥
garlic powder	9	1.7	0.5	0.3	0	♥♥♥
ginger, ground	6	1.1	0.2	0.2	0.1	♥♥♥
horseradish, 1 tbsp	7	1.2	0.2	0.5	0.1	♥♥♥
mace, ground	8	0.6	0.1	0.3	0.6	♥♥♥
marjoram, dried	2	0.2	0.1	0.2	0	♥♥♥
mustard seed	15	0.7	0.8	0.5	1	♥♥♥
nutmeg, ground	12	0.6	0.1	0.5	0.8	♥♥♥

 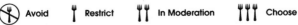

Avoid   Restrict   In Moderation   Choose

Food	Cal	Net Carb	Protein	Fiber	Total Fat	Advice
onion powder	8	1.8	0.2	0.1	0	♟♟♟
oregano, dried	3	0.2	0.1	0.4	0.1	♟♟♟
oregano, dried, ground	6	0.4	0.2	0.8	0.2	♟♟♟
paprika	6	0.4	0.3	0.8	0.3	♟♟♟
parsley, dried	1	0.1	0.1	0.1	0	♟♟♟
peppermint, fresh, 2 tbsp	2	0.2	0.1	0.3	0	♟♟♟
poppy seed	15	0.4	0.5	0.3	1.3	♟♟♟
poultry seasoning, 1 tbsp	11	2	0.4	0.4	0.3	♟♟♟
pumpkin pie spice, 1 tbsp	19	3.1	0.3	0.8	0.7	♟♟♟
rosemary, dried	4	0.3	0.1	0.5	0.2	♟♟♟
rosemary, fresh, 1 tbsp	2	0.2	0.1	0.2	0.1	♟♟♟
saffron	2	0.5	0.1	0	0	♟♟♟
sage, ground	2	0.1	0.1	0.3	0.1	♟♟♟
salt	0	0	0	0	0	♟♟♟
savory, ground	4	0.4	0.1	0.6	0.1	♟♟♟
spearmint, dried	1	0.2	0.1	0.1	0	♟♟♟
spearmint, fresh, 2 tbsp	5	0.2	0.4	0.8	0.1	♟♟♟

*contains sugar alcohols

Food	Cal	Net Carb	Protein	Fiber	Total Fat	Advice
tarragon, dried	2	0.3	0.1	0	0	▓▓▓
thyme, dried	3	0.2	0.1	0.4	0.1	▓▓▓
thyme, fresh	1	0.1	0	0.1	0	▓▓▓
turmeric, ground	8	0.9	0.2	0.5	0.2	▓▓▓
vanilla extract	12	0.5	0	0	0	▓▓▓
vanilla extract, imitation, no alcohol	2	0.6	0	0	0	▓▓▓
vanilla extract, imitation, w/alcohol	10	0.1	0	0	0	▓▓▓
white pepper	7	1.1	0.3	0.6	0.1	▓▓▓
Syrups						
chocolate, 2 tbsp	109	24.4	0.8	1	0.4	⊘
chocolate fudge, 2 tbsp	133	22.8	1.8	1.1	3.4	⊘
chocolate, lite, Hershey's, 2 tbsp	50	11.9	0.3	0	0.2	⊘
grenadine, 1 tbsp	53	13.3	0	0	0	⊘
malt, 2 tbsp	153	34.2	3	0	0	⊘
maple syrup, 1 tbsp	52	13.4	0	0	0	⊘
maple syrup, sugar-free, Joseph's, 1/4 cup (60ml)*	35	0	0	0	0	▓▓▓
sugar-free, low-carb, Atkins, 1 tbsp	0	0	0	0	0	▓▓▓

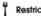 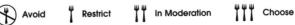

⊘ Avoid   ▓ Restrict   ▓▓ In Moderation   ▓▓▓ Choose

Seafood

THE GOOD NEWS IS THAT FISH IS ONE OF THE BEST FOODS ON THE planet. There has always been one principle upon which everyone in the diet wars could agree: the more fish the better.

Here's the bad news: our fish supply is becoming increasingly contaminated with chemicals, heavy metals, and antibiotics.

Ocean fish now often contains mercury. The Environmental Working Group (EWG) lists fourteen types of fish on its "do not eat if pregnant" list because of mercury content—another nine are listed as "eat no more than once a month." Four types of fish—canned albacore tuna, grouper, sea bass, and bluefish—are especially troublesome. The EWG reports that canned albacore has twice as much mercury as the FDA estimates, and three times the mercury levels of light tuna.

Then farm-raised fish should be fine, right? Think again. The EWG reports that farmed salmon sold in U.S. grocery stores is the most PCB-contaminated protein source in the domestic food supply. PCBs, or polychlorinated biphenyls, are nasty chemical toxins you don't want to be ingesting at all.

What to do? Well, I rarely order farm-raised salmon from restaurants anymore. I do, however, eat *wild* Alaskan salmon, particularly red sockeye. I buy my fish from Vital Choice (www.VitalChoice.com), where it's stringently tested for contaminants, metals, and PCBs. And I'm careful to check the advisory warnings on the Environmental Working Group website, www.ewg.org.

Oh, and one more thing: stock up on sardines. Because these are so low on the food chain, they don't seem to accumulate much of the bad stuff. Plus, they're cheap, easy to find, and a wonderful source of both protein and omega-3 fats. They're the original health food in a can.

SEAFOOD						
Food	Cal	Net Carb	Protein	Fiber	Total Fat	Advice
Canned Fish						
anchovy, in oil, 2 oz	94	0	13	0	4.4	🍴🍴🍴
cod, Atlantic, 3 oz	89	0	19.4	0	0.7	🍴🍴🍴
mackerel, 3 oz	132	0	19.8	0	5.4	🍴🍴🍴
salmon, w/o salt, 3 oz	118	0	16.8	0	5.1	🍴🍴🍴
sardine, in oil, 3 oz	177	0	21	0	9.9	🍴🍴🍴
tuna, in water, 3 oz						
light	99	0	21.7	0	0.7	🍴🍴🍴
light, w/o salt	99	0	21.7	0	0.7	🍴🍴🍴
white	109	0	20.1	0	2.5	🍴🍴🍴
white, w/o salt	109	0	20.1	0	2.5	🍴🍴🍴
Canned Shellfish						
clam, 3 oz	126	0	21.7	0	1.7	🍴🍴🍴
crab, blue, 3 oz	84	0	17.4	0	1.1	🍴🍴🍴
oyster, eastern, 3 oz	48	2.7	4.9	0	1.7	🍴🍴🍴
shrimp, 4.5 oz	154	1.3	29.5	0	2.5	🍴🍴🍴

 Avoid   Restrict    In Moderation   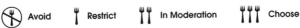 Choose

Food	Cal	Net Carb	Protein	Fiber	Total Fat	Advice
Caviar and Roe, 1 oz						
caviar, black and red, granular	71	1.1	7	0	5.1	🍴🍴🍴
roe, baked, broiled, or grilled	58	0.5	8.1	0	2.3	🍴🍴🍴
Fresh Fish, Baked, Broiled, or Grilled unless noted, 3 oz serving						
bass, freshwater	124	0	20.6	0	4	🍴🍴🍴
bass, striped	105	0	19.3	0	2.5	🍴🍴🍴
bluefish	135	0	21.8	0	4.6	🍴🍴🍴
burbot	98	0	21.1	0	0.9	🍴🍴🍴
butterfish	159	0	18.8	0	8.7	🍴🍴🍴
carp	138	0	19.4	0	6.1	🍴🍴🍴
catfish, channel, breaded and fried	195	6.2	15.4	0.6	11.3	🚫🍴
catfish, channel, farmed	129	0	15.9	0	6.8	🍴🍴
cisco, smoked	150	0	13.9	0	10.1	🍴
cod, Atlantic	89	0	19.4	0	0.7	🍴🍴🍴
cod, Pacific	89	0	19.5	0	0.7	🍴🍴🍴
croaker, Atlantic, breaded and fried	188	6.1	15.5	0.3	10.8	🚫🍴
cusk	95	0	20.7	0	0.8	🍴🍴🍴
dolphinfish	93	0	20.2	0	0.8	🍴🍴🍴
drum, freshwater	130	0	19.1	0	5.4	🍴🍴🍴

ND = No Data

Food	Cal	Net Carb	Protein	Fiber	Total Fat	Advice
eel	201	0	20.1	0	12.7	⑁⑁⑁
flatfish (flounder and sole species)	99	0	20.5	0	1.3	⑁⑁⑁
grouper	100	0	21.1	0	1.1	⑁⑁⑁
haddock	95	0	20.6	0	0.8	⑁⑁⑁
halibut, Atlantic and Pacific	119	0	22.7	0	2.5	⑁⑁⑁
herring, Atlantic	173	0	19.6	0	9.9	⑁⑁⑁
herring, Pacific	212	0	17.9	0	15.1	⑁⑁⑁
ling	94	0	20.7	0	0.7	⑁⑁⑁
lingcod	93	0	19.2	0	1.2	⑁⑁⑁
mackerel, Atlantic	223	0	20.3	0	15.1	⑁⑁⑁
mackerel, king	114	0	22.1	0	2.2	⑁⑁⑁
monkfish	82	0	15.8	0	1.7	⑁⑁⑁
mullet, striped	128	0	21.1	0	4.1	⑁⑁⑁
perch	99	0	21.1	0	1	⑁⑁⑁
pike, northern	96	0	21	0	0.8	⑁⑁⑁
pike, walleye	101	0	20.9	0	1.3	⑁⑁⑁
pollock, Atlantic	100	0	21.2	0	1.1	⑁⑁⑁

 Avoid   Restrict   In Moderation   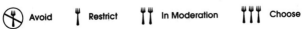 Choose

Food	Cal	Net Carb	Protein	Fiber	Total Fat	Advice
pollock, walleye	96	0	20	0	1	ŤŤŤ
pompano, Florida	179	0	20.1	0	10.3	ŤŤŤ
pout, ocean	87	0	18.1	0	1	ŤŤŤ
rockfish, Pacific	103	0	20.4	0	1.7	ŤŤŤ
roughy, orange	76	0	16	0	0.8	ŤŤŤ
sablefish	212	0	14.6	0	16.7	ŤŤŤ
salmon						
Atlantic, farmed	175	0	18.8	0	10.5	ŤŤŤ
Atlantic, wild	155	0	21.6	0	6.9	ŤŤŤ
chinook	196	0	21.9	0	11.4	ŤŤŤ
coho, farmed	151	0	20.7	0	7	ŤŤŤ
sockeye	184	0	23.2	0	9.3	ŤŤŤ
scup	115	0	20.6	0	3	ŤŤŤ
sea bass	105	0	20.1	0	2.2	ŤŤŤ
seatrout	113	0	18.2	0	3.9	ŤŤŤ
shad, American	214	0	18.5	0	15	ŤŤŤ
sheepshead	107	0	22.1	0	1.4	ŤŤŤ
snapper	109	0	22.4	0	1.5	ŤŤŤ
sturgeon	115	0	17.6	0	4.4	ŤŤŤ

Food	Cal	Net Carb	Protein	Fiber	Total Fat	Advice
swordfish	132	0	21.6	0	4.4	ϯϯϯ
trout	162	0	22.6	0	7.2	ϯϯϯ
trout, rainbow, farmed	144	0	20.6	0	6.1	ϯϯϯ
trout, rainbow, wild	128	0	19.5	0	5	ϯϯϯ
tuna, 3 oz serving						
bluefin	156	0	25.4	0	5.3	ϯϯϯ
skipjack	112	0	24	0	1.1	ϯϯϯ
yellowfin	118	0	25.5	0	1	ϯϯϯ
whitefish	146	0	20.8	0	6.4	ϯϯϯ
whiting	99	0	20	0	1.4	ϯϯϯ
wolffish, Atlantic	105	0	19.1	0	2.6	ϯϯϯ
yellowtail	159	0	25.2	0	5.7	ϯϯϯ
Fresh Shellfish, Boiled, Steamed, or Poached unless noted, 3 oz serving unless noted						
abalone, fried	161	9.4	16.7	0	5.8	ϯϯϯ
clam, breaded and fried	172	8.8	12.1	0	9.5	ϯϯϯ
clam	126	4.4	21.7	0	1.7	ϯϯϯ
conch, baked or broiled	66	0.9	13.4	0	0.6	ϯϯϯ

 Avoid   Restrict   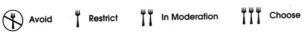 In Moderation   Choose

Food	Cal	Net Carb	Protein	Fiber	Total Fat	Advice
crab						
Alaska king	82	0	16.5	0	1.3	♟♟♟
Alaska king, imitation, made from surimi	87	8.7	10.2	0	1.1	♟♟♟
blue	87	0	17.2	0	1.5	♟♟♟
Dungeness	94	0.8	19	0	1.1	♟♟♟
Dungeness, 1 crab	140	1.2	28.4	0	1.6	♟♟♟
queen	98	0	20.2	0	1.3	♟♟♟
lobster, northern	83	1.1	17.4	0	0.5	♟♟♟
mussel, blue	146	6.3	20.2	0	3.8	♟♟♟
octopus, common	139	3.7	25.4	0	1.8	♟♟♟
oyster						
eastern, breaded and fried	167	9.9	7.5	0	10.7	♟♟♟
eastern, farmed, baked, broiled, or grilled	67	6.2	6	0	1.8	♟♟♟
eastern, wild	116	6.7	12	0	4.2	♟♟♟
Pacific	139	8.4	16.1	0	3.9	♟♟♟
scallop (bay and sea), steamed	95	0	19.7	0	1.2	♟♟♟
scallop, breaded and fried	183	8.6	15.4	0	9.3	♟♟♟
scallop, imitation, made from surimi	84	9	10.9	0	0.4	♟♟♟

Food	Cal	Net Carb	Protein	Fiber	Total Fat	Advice
shrimp						
4 large shrimp	22	0	4.6	0	0.2	♟♟♟
10 shrimp	38	0.3	7.4	0	0.6	♟♟♟
breaded and fried, 4 large shrimp	73	3.3	6.4	0.1	3.7	⊗
imitation, made from surimi	86	7.8	10.5	0	1.3	♟♟
squid, fried	149	6.6	15.3	0	6.4	⊗

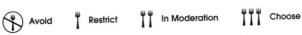

⊗ Avoid   ♟ Restrict   ♟♟ In Moderation   ♟♟♟ Choose

Snacks

RATING THESE FOODS—IF YOU CAN CALL THEM THAT—IS A TRICKY business. Practically every day a new study reveals just how bad for us sugar really is. I wouldn't be surprised if, in fifty years, the sugar industry experiences exactly the same public-relations nightmare that the tobacco industry is experiencing today. Sugar depresses the immune system, depletes important minerals from the body, causes all sorts of metabolic issues, contributes to weight gain and diabetes, and is now associated with at least four different kinds of cancer.

That said, I've tried to recommend the snacks that are the "least bad"—either in terms of carbs or calories. That doesn't mean they're good. But it also doesn't mean you can never ever eat the snacks that got an "Avoid" rating—just be aware that their carbohydrate and calorie content is very high, and they may be difficult to fit into your low-carb plan.

Some of the low-carb candies—like Atkins Endulge and its many imitators—use sugar alcohols for sweetening. I think sugar alcohols are far from the worst thing you can eat—but I also worry that they are being used more than is justified by our still-limited knowledge of how they work. One of them—maltitol—has already been shown to have a higher glycemic impact than was previously thought, especially in sensitive diabetics. So even the best of the low carb candies received only a "Restrict" rating from me. And having a low carb count doesn't necessarily mean that they have a low *calorie* count. The best of them taste so darn good they might well be as addictive for some people as regular candy. Consumer beware.

SNACKS

Food	Cal	Net Carb	Protein	Fiber	Total Fat	Glycemic Load	Advice
Candy							
After Eight Mints, 5 pieces	147	30.6	0.9	0.9	5.6	ND	
butterscotch candies, 3 pieces	63	14.5	0	0	0.5	ND	⊺
caramel candies, 1 piece	39	7.7	0.5	0.1	0.8	ND	⊺
peanuts, milk chocolate-coated, 10 pieces	208	17.9	5.2	1.9	13.4	ND	
raisins, milk chocolate-coated, 10 pieces	39	6.4	0.4	0.4	1.5	ND	⊺
fudge, chocolate, 1 piece	70	12.7	0.4	0.3	1.8	ND	⊺
fudge, vanilla, 1 piece	65	14	0.2	0	0.9	ND	⊺
goobers, 1/4 cup	210	17.5	5.6	2.5	13.7	ND	
gumdrops, 10 pieces	143	35.1	0	0	0	ND	
gumdrops, sugar-free, Estee, 11 pieces*	110	5	0	ND	0	ND	⊺
gummy bears, 10 pieces	87	21.8	0	0	0	ND	⊺
gummy bears, sugar-free, Estee, 17 pieces*	110	0	3	ND	0	ND	⊺
hard candy, peppermint, 3 pieces	59	14.7	0	ND	0	Med.	⊺
hard candy, sugar-free, Fifty 50, mint, 4 pieces*	30	0	0	0	0	ND	⊺
jellybeans, 10 small pieces	41	10.3	0	0	0	Low	⊺

*contains sugar alcohols

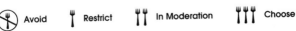

 Avoid   ⊺ Restrict   In Moderation   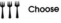 Choose

Food	Cal	Net Carb	Protein	Fiber	Total Fat	Glycemic Load	Advice
jellybeans, sugar-free, Estee, 26 pieces*	110	3	0	ND	0	ND	⍦
M&M's, milk chocolate, 1 package (1.69 oz)	236	33	2.1	1.2	10.1	ND	⊗
marshmallows, 1/2 cup miniatures	80	20.3	0.5	0	0.1	ND	⍦
Peanut Butter Cups, Reese's, 2 cups (1.6 oz)	232	23.3	4.6	1.6	13.7	ND	⊗
Peanut Butter Cups, fructose sweetened, Estee, 5 pieces	200	18	5	1	12	ND	⊗
Peanut Butter Cups, low-carb, Atkins Endulge, 3 cups*	160	2	3	0	13	ND	⍦
Peppermint Patty, York, 1 patty (1.5 oz)	165	33.9	0.9	0.9	3.1	ND	⊗
Peppermint Patties, low-carb, Russell Stover, 2 pieces*	130	0	1	1	7	ND	⍦
Peppermint Patties, sugar-free, Sorbee, 6 pieces*	190	4	3	1	14	ND	⍦
Raisinets, 1 package (1.58 oz)	185	32	2.1	ND	7.2	ND	⊗
Reese's Pieces, 1 package (1.63 oz)	229	26.1	5.7	1.4	11.4	ND	⊗
Skittles, 1 package (2.3 oz)	263	58.9	0.1	0	2.8	High	⊗
Starburst, 5 pieces	99	21.1	0.1	0	2.1	ND	⍦
Truffles, sugar-free, Sorbee, 5 pieces*	180	4	2	1	14	ND	⍦
Twizzlers, 4 pieces from 5 oz pack	133	30.3	1	0	0.9	ND	⊗
Wafer Crisps, low-carb, Atkins Endulge, 2 bars*	120	4	4	3	9	ND	⍦
candy bars							
3 Musketeers, 1 bar (1.813 oz)	212	38.3	1.6	0.9	6.6	Med.	⊗

*contains sugar alcohols

ND = No Data

Food	Cal	Net Carb	Protein	Fiber	Total Fat	Glycemic Load	Advice
Hershey, milk chocolate, 1 bar (0.6 oz)	90	9	1	1	5	Med.	
Kit Kat, 1 bar (1.5 oz)	217	26.2	2.7	0.8	11.4	Med.	
Mars Almond, 1 bar (1.76 oz)	234	30.4	4.1	1	11.5	Med.	
Milky Way, 1 bar (1.9 oz)	228	37.8	2.4	0.9	8.7	Med.	
Nestlè Crunch, 1 bar (1.4 oz)	209	25.1	2.4	1	10.5	Med.	
Snickers, 1 bar (2 oz)	273	32.4	4.6	1.4	14	Med.	
Special Dark Chocolate Bar, 1 bar (1.45 oz)	218	21.7	2.3	2.7	13.3	Med.	
Twix, 2 bars (2.06 oz)	289	37.4	2.7	0.6	14.2	Med.	
chocolate bars, low-carb							
Atkins Endulge, low-carb, 1 bar*	150	2	1	3	12	Low	
almond, Fifty 50, w/out added sugar, 7 pieces*	180	11	4	1	13	Low	
Caramel Nut Chew, low-carb, Atkins Endulge, 1 bar*	140	2	6	2	9	Med.	
crunch, Fifty 50, w/out added sugar, 7 pieces*	140	10	3	1	9	Low	
dark chocolate, Sorbee Zero Sugar, no sugar, 1/2 bar*	180	3	2	6	12	Low	
milk chocolate, Fifty 50, w/out added sugar, 7 pieces*	180	11	4	1	13	Low	
milk chocolate bar, Sorbee Zero Sugar, no sugar, 1/2 bar*	190	0	3	1	13	Low	
milk chocolate w/almonds, Estee, fructose sweetened, 7 squares	230	16	4	0	17	Low	

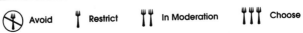

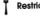 Avoid   Restrict   In Moderation   Choose

Food	Cal	Net Carb	Protein	Fiber	Total Fat	Glycemic Load	Advice
milk chocolate w/peanuts bar, Sorbee Zero Sugar, no sugar, 1/2 bar*	200	1	4	1	14	Low	🚫🍴
Chips							
corn chips, Fritos, 1 oz (32 chips)	160	14	2	1	10	Low	🚫🍴
low-carb, Atkins Crunchers, BBQ, 1 package	100	4	13	4	3	ND	🍴
low-carb, Atkins Crunchers, original, 1 package	90	4	13	4	3	ND	🍴
low-carb, Atkins Crunchers, sour cream and onion, 1 package	100	5	12	3	4	ND	🍴
multigrain chips, Sunchips, 1 oz (11 chips)	140	17	2	2	6	ND	🍴
potato chips							
potato chips, 1 oz	152	13.7	2	1.3	9.8	Low	🚫🍴
Lay's Baked, 1 oz (11 chips)	110	21	2	2	1.5	Med.	🚫🍴
tortilla chips							
regular, 1 oz	142	16	2	1.8	7.4	Med.	🍴
Doritos, 1 oz (12 chips)	140	16	2	1	8	Low	🍴
Doritos Baked, 1 oz (15 chips)	120	19	2	2	3.5	ND	🍴
low-carb, CarbSense Soy Multigrain, 18 chips	145	8	4	4	9	ND	🍴🍴
nacho, 1 oz	141	16.2	2.2	1.5	7.3	Med.	🍴
Tostitos Baked, 1 oz (9 chips)	110	22	2	2	1	ND	🍴

*contains sugar alcohols

Food	Cal	Net Carb	Protein	Fiber	Total Fat	Glycemic Load	Advice
Crackers							
cheese, 5 small squares	25	2.8	0.5	0.1	1.3	ND	
matzo, plain, 1 serving	111	22.6	2.8	0.8	0.4	ND	
matzo, whole-wheat, 1 serving	98	18.8	3.7	3.3	0.4	ND	
melba toast, 2 pieces	39	7.1	1.2	0.6	0.3	Low	
melba toast, wheat, 2 pieces	37	6.9	1.3	0.7	0.2	Low	
oyster crackers, 1/2 cup	98	15.4	2.1	0.7	2.7	ND	
Ritz, 1 serving (16 grams)	79	10	1.2	0.3	3.7	ND	
saltines, 4 crackers	104	16.5	2.2	0.7	2.8	ND	
Triscuits, 6 crackers	130	16	3	3	5	ND	
wheat, 6 crackers	57	7.3	1	0.5	2.5	Low	
Wheat Thins, 1 serving	136	19.1	2.4	0.9	5.8	ND	
Fruit Snacks							
banana chips, 3 oz	441	43.1	2	6.5	28.6	ND	
fruit roll-ups, 2 rolls	104	23.9	0	ND	1	High	
fruit leather, 1 bar	81	17.3	0.4	0.8	1.2	Med.	
Granola Bars, 1 bar							
chocolate chip, Quaker Chewy	120	20	1	1	4	ND	

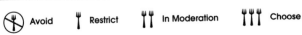

Avoid   Restrict   In Moderation   Choose

Food	Cal	Net Carb	Protein	Fiber	Total Fat	Glycemic Load	Advice
oatmeal raisin, Quaker Chewy Wholesome Favorites	110	21	1	1	2	ND	🍴
Meat							
beef jerky, 1 piece	82	1.8	6.6	0.4	5.1	ND	🍴🍴🍴
beef sticks, smoked, 1 stick	110	1.1	4.3	ND	9.9	ND	🍴🍴🍴
pork skins, 1 oz	155	0	17.4	0	8.9	ND	🍴🍴
Miscellaneous Snacks							
Cheetos, 1 cup	150	15	2	1	9	ND	🍴
Chex Mix, 2 oz	242	33.9	6.3	3.2	9.9	ND	🍴
cornnuts, 1 oz	126	18.4	2.4	2	4.4	ND	🍴
Just the Cheese snack bars, low-carb, 1 bar	75	0.5	5	0	6.5	ND	🍴🍴🍴
Just the Cheese snacks, low-carb, 1 oz	150	3	10	0	13	ND	🍴🍴🍴
oriental mix, 1 oz	143	10.9	4.9	3.7	7.3	ND	🍴
trail mix, chocolate chips, salted nuts, and seeds, 1 cup	707	65.6	20.7	ND	46.6	ND	🍴
Nutrition/Sports Bars, 1 bar							
All In One Bar	180	15	15	5	5	ND	🍴🍴
Atkins Advantage Almond Brownie Bar	220	2	21	7	8	ND	🍴🍴🍴
Balance Bar	200	22	14	0	6	ND	🍴
Balance Bar Gold	210	22	15	1	6	ND	🍴

*contains sugar alcohols

Food	Cal	Net Carb	Protein	Fiber	Total Fat	Glycemic Load	Advice
Carb Options Bar*	200	3	16	1	8	ND	In Moderation
Clif Bar							
chocolate chip peanut crunch	250	38	11	5	6	ND	Avoid
Builder's Bar	270	26	20	4	8	ND	Avoid
Luna Bar	180	25	10	2	4	ND	Avoid
Luna Glow Bar*	140	3	8	1	7	ND	Choose
Deliciously Slim Protein Bar*	200	2	20	1	6	ND	Restrict
Doctor's CarbRite Diet Sugar-Free Bar, chocolate brownie*	185	2.5	20.5	0	3.3	ND	In Moderation
Ketogenics Bar*	280	1	5	2	20	ND	Avoid
Met-Rx Big 100 Bar	360	49	27	2	5	High	Avoid
Met-Rx Protein Plus Bar	320	28	34	1	8	High	Avoid
Nutribar*	250	27	13	4	8	ND	Avoid
Power Bars							
Harvest	240	41	7	4	4	ND	Avoid
Harvest Dipped	250	43	7	2	5	ND	Avoid
Performance	230	42	10	3	2	ND	Avoid
Pria	110	16	5	ND	3	ND	In Moderation
Pria Carb Select*	170	2	10	2	8	ND	Choose

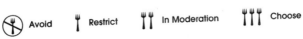

 Avoid   Restrict   In Moderation   Choose

Food	Cal	Net Carb	Protein	Fiber	Total Fat	Glycemic Load	Advice
Protein Plus	290	36	24	1	5	ND	(fork in circle)
Protein Plus Carb Select*	260	2	22	1	7	ND	(fork in circle)
Protein Plus, layered	220	25	15	1	6	ND	(fork in circle)
Protein Plus, sugar-free*	170	1	16	1	4	ND	2 forks
Slim Fast Meal Bar	220	32	8	2	5	Low	(fork in circle)
Slim Fast Snack Bar	120	22	1	0	3.5	Low	(fork in circle)
Slim Fast Succeed Snack Bar*	120	3	6	1	3	Low	3 forks
Snickers Marathon	220	25	13	2	7	ND	(fork in circle)
Tiger's Milk Bar	150	17	6	1	7	ND	(fork in circle)
Zone Perfect Bar	210	22	16	0	7	ND	(fork in circle)
Nutrition/Sports Shakes							
Atkins Advantage Shake, powder, 2 scoops (34 grams)*	140	3	15	5	4	ND	3 forks
Atkins Shake, 1 can	170	1	20	3	9	ND	3 forks
Atkins Shake, powder, 2 scoops (43 grams)	170	2	23	0	8	ND	3 forks
Boost, 1 can (8 fl oz)	240	41	10	0	4	ND	(fork in circle)
Ensure shakes, 1 can, 8 fl oz							
regular	250	39	9	1	6	Med.	(fork in circle)
Fiber w/FOS	250	39	9	3	6	Med.	(fork in circle)

*contains sugar alcohols

Food	Cal	Net Carb	Protein	Fiber	Total Fat	Glycemic Load	Advice
Plus	350	49	13	1	11	High	
Glucerna, 1 can (8 fl oz)*	220	20	10	3	8.5	Low	
Slim Fast, 1 can (11 fl oz)	220	35	10	5	2.5	Med.	
Slim Fast Low-Carb Diet Meal Shake, 1 can	190	2	20	2	9	ND	
Snapple a Day Meal Replacement Shake, 1 can (11.5 fl oz)	210	38	7	5	0	ND	
Popcorn							
air-popped, 1 cup	31	5	0.96	1.2	0.3	Low	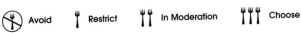
microwave butter lover's, Act, 2 tbsp, unpopped	170	13	2	3	12	Low	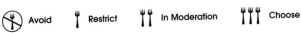
oil-popped, 1 cup	55	5.2	0.99	1.1	3.1	Low	
Pretzels							
pretzels, regular, 1 oz	108	21.7	2.6	0.8	1	Med.	
soft pretzel, 1 large	483	96.8	11.7	2.4	4.4	ND	
whole-wheat pretzels, 1 oz	103	20.8	3.2	2.2	0.7	Med.	
Rice Cakes							
brown rice, 1 cake	35	6.9	0.7	0.4	0.3	Low	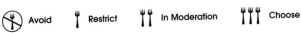
caramel corn, apple cinnamon, Quaker, 1 cake	50	12	1	ND	0	Low	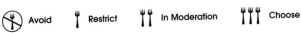
white cheddar, Quaker, 1 cake	45	8	1	ND	0.5	Low	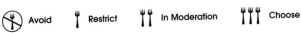

 Avoid   Restrict   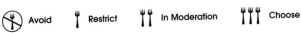 In Moderation   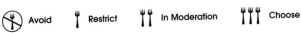 Choose

Vegetables

LET'S GET ONE THING CLEAR RIGHT OFF THE BAT: ALL VEGETABLES are good. Period.

Now, okay, maybe I need to clarify a bit (especially since the most consumed "vegetables" in America are lettuce, ketchup, and french fries). I'm talking anything with a leaf. I'm talking anything that has a crunch. I'm talking anything that's green, red, or orange. Get the drift? I'm definitely not talking french fries.

This may seem self-evident, but it's not. There's a lot of confusion about certain starchy vegetables that have a high glycemic index (carrots, for example). In the introductory discussion of the glycemic index and glycemic load (page 11), I tell you why the glycemic index is *not* important, and why you should instead pay attention to the glycemic load. Bottom line: carrots are fine.

Potatoes, however, are not. They have a high glycemic index *and* load. Corn is up there too. So I'd be careful loading up on the really starchy veggies. When a swallow of potatoes hits your esophagus, all your body sees is a big ball of sugar. Stick to the green leafy stuff.

Vegetables are loaded with fiber, phytonutrients, vitamins, antioxidants, and all that good stuff. Shop for color. The more the better.

Plus, vegetables fill you up like crazy. Even during the low-fat craze of the 1980s, I'd often recommend that my clients steam a huge plate of broccoli and sweet red onions, then throw a slab of butter on the mix and enjoy. Of course, in those days they'd look at me, horrified, and say, "Butter? Are you crazy? What about all that *fat?*"

Relax. Butter is a good fat, and anything that makes a big plate of vegetables more palatable for you is a friend of mine.

VEGETABLES

Food	Cal	Net Carb	Protein	Fiber	Total Fat	Glycemic Load	Advice
alfalfa sprouts, raw, 1 cup	10	0.5	1.3	0.8	0.2	ND	¶¶¶
artichoke, boiled, 1/2 cup	42	4.9	2.9	4.5	0.1	Low	¶¶¶
asparagus, cooked, 1/2 cup	20	1.9	2.2	1.8	0.2	ND	¶¶¶
bamboo shoots, canned, 1 cup	25	2.4	2.3	1.8	0.5	ND	¶¶¶
bean sprouts, crunchy, 1/2 cup	24	0	2	1	1	ND	¶¶¶
beans (*see* Legumes)							
beet greens, cooked, 1 cup	39	3.7	3.7	4.2	0.3	ND	¶¶¶
beets, canned, 1 cup, sliced	53	9.4	1.6	2.9	0.2	Low	¶¶
broccoli raab, cooked, 1 serving (85 grams)	28	0.3	3.3	2.4	0.5	ND	¶¶¶
broccoli, cooked, 1 cup, chopped	27	3	1.9	2.6	0.3	Low	¶¶¶
broccoli, raw, 1 cup, chopped	30	3.5	2.5	2.3	0.3	Low	¶¶¶
broccosprouts, 1/2 cup	5	0	1	1	0	ND	¶¶¶
brussel sprouts, cooked, 1/2 cup	28	3.5	2	2	0.4	ND	¶¶¶
cabbage							
common, cooked, 1/2 cup, shredded	16	2	0.8	1.4	0.3	Low	¶¶¶
napa, cooked, 1 cup	13	2.4	1.2		0.2	Low	¶¶¶
pak-choi, cooked, 1 cup, shredded	20	1.3	2.7	1.7	0.3	Low	¶¶¶
red, raw, 1 cup, shredded	22	3.7	1	1.5	0.1	Low	¶¶¶

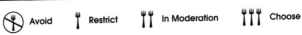 Avoid   Restrict   In Moderation   Choose

Food	Cal	Net Carb	Protein	Fiber	Total Fat	Glycemic Load	Advice
carrot juice, 1 cup	94	20	2.2	1.9	0.4	Low	⍾
carrots, baby, raw, 1 large baby carrot	5	0.9	0.1	0.3	0	Low	⍾⍾⍾
carrots, cooked, 1/2 cup, sliced	27	4.1	0.6	2.3	0.1	Low	⍾⍾⍾
carrots, raw, 1 cup, sliced	50	8	1.1	3.7	0.3	Low	⍾⍾⍾
cauliflower, cooked, 1/2 cup, pieces	14	0.9	1.1	1.7	0.3	Low	⍾⍾⍾
cauliflower, raw, 1 cup	25	2.8	2	2.5	0.1	Low	⍾⍾⍾
celery, raw, 1 cup, diced	17	1.7	0.8	1.9	0.2	Low	⍾⍾⍾
chayote, cooked, 1 cup, pieces	38	3.6	1	4.5	0.8	ND	⍾⍾⍾
chicory greens, raw, 1 cup, chopped	41	1.3	3.1	7.2	0.5	ND	⍾⍾⍾
chives, raw, 1 tbsp, chopped	1	0	0.1	0.1	0	ND	⍾⍾⍾
collards, cooked, 1 cup, chopped	49	4	4	5.3	0.7	ND	⍾⍾⍾
corn, cooked, 1 cup	177	36.6	5.4	4.6	2.1	High	🚫
corn on the cob, cooked, 1 ear of kernels	59	12.3	2	1.8	0.5	Med.	⍾⍾
cucumber, raw, 1/2 cup, sliced	8	1.6	0.3	0.3	0.1	Low	⍾⍾⍾
dandelion greens, cooked, 1 cup	35	3.7	2.1	3	0.6	ND	⍾⍾⍾
eggplant, cooked, 1 cup, cubed	35	6.1	0.8	2.5	0.2	ND	⍾⍾⍾
endive, raw, 1/2 cup, chopped	4	0	0.3	0.8	0.1	ND	⍾⍾⍾
fennel, raw, 1 cup, sliced	27	3.6	1.1	2.7	0	ND	⍾⍾⍾

ND = No Data

Food	Cal	Net Carb	Protein	Fiber	Total Fat	Glycemic Load	Advice
gourd, dishcloth, cooked, 1 cup, pieces	100	25.5	1.2	ND	0.6	ND	
gourd, white-flowered, cooked, 1 cup, cubed	22	5.4	0.9	ND	0	ND	
grape leaves, canned, 1 leaf	3	0.5	0.2	ND	0.1	ND	
green snap beans, frozen, 1 cup	41	5.9	2.2	3.5	0.3	ND	
hearts of palm, canned, 1 cup	41	3.3	3.7	3.5	0.9	ND	
kale, cooked, 1 cup, chopped	36	4.7	2.5	2.6	0.5	ND	
leeks, cooked, 1/4 cup	8	1.7	0.2	0.3	0.1	ND	
lemon grass, raw, 1 tbsp	5	1.2	0.1	ND	0	ND	
lettuce							
butterhead, 1 cup, chopped	7	0.6	0.7	0.6	0.1	Low	
green leaf, 1/2 cup, shredded	4	0.4	0.4	0.4	0	Low	
iceberg, 1 cup, chopped	6	0.6	0.5	0.6	0.1	Low	
red leaf, 1 cup, shredded	4	0.3	0.4	0.3	0.1	Low	
romaine, 1/2 cup, shredded	5	0.3	0.3	0.6	0.1	Low	
lotus root, cooked, 1/2 cup	40	7.7	1	1.9	0	ND	
mushroom							
1 cup boiled, pieces	44	4.9	3.4	3.4	0.7	ND	
1 cup raw, sliced	15	1.5	2.2	0.8	0.2	ND	

 Avoid    Restrict   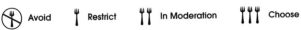 In Moderation   Choose

Food	Cal	Net Carb	Protein	Fiber	Total Fat	Glycemic Load	Advice
crimini, raw, 1 piece	3	0.5	0.4	0.1	0	ND	ŸŸŸ
oyster, raw, 1 large	55	5.6	6.1	3.6	0.8	ND	ŸŸŸ
portabella, raw (100 grams)	26	3.6	2.5	1.5	0.2	ND	ŸŸŸ
shiitake, cooked, 1 cup, pieces	80	17.7	2.3	3	0.3	ND	ŸŸŸ
straw, canned, 1 cup	58	3.9	7	4.5	1.2	ND	ŸŸŸ
mustard greens, cooked, 1 cup, chopped	21	0.1	3.2	2.8	0.3	ND	ŸŸŸ
okra, cooked, 1/2 cup, sliced	18	1.6	1.5	2	0.1	ND	ŸŸŸ
onion							
boiled, whole, 1 medium	41	8.24	1.3	1.3	0.2	ND	ŸŸŸ
boiled, 1 cup, chopped	92	18.4	2.9	2.9	0.4	ND	ŸŸ
raw, 1 cup, sliced	48	10	1.1	1.6	0.1	ND	ŸŸŸ
scallions, raw, 1 cup, chopped	32	4.7	1.8	2.6	0.2	ND	ŸŸŸ
sweet, raw, 1 serving (148 grams)	47	9.9	1.2	1.3	0.1	ND	ŸŸŸ
young green, raw, 1 tbsp	2	0.1	0.1	0.2	0	ND	ŸŸŸ
parsley, raw, 1 tbsp	1	0.1	0.1	0.1	0	ND	ŸŸŸ
parsnips, cooked, 1/2 cup, sliced	55	10.5	1	2.8	0.2	Med.	ŸŸŸ
peapods, cooked, 1 cup	83	9.4	5.6	5	0.6	ND	ŸŸŸ
peas, green, cooked, 1 cup	134	16.2	8.6	8.8	0.4	Low	ŸŸ

Food	Cal	Net Carb	Protein	Fiber	Total Fat	Glycemic Load	Advice
peppers							
banana, raw, 1 cup	33	2.4	2.1	4.2	0.6	Low	Choose
hot chili, green, raw, 1 pepper	18	3.6	0.9	0.7	0.1	Low	Choose
hot chili, red, raw, 1 pepper	19	3	0.8	0.7	0.5	Low	Choose
hot chili, sundried, 1 pepper	2	0.3	0.1	0.1	0	Low	Choose
jalapeno, raw, 1 pepper	4	0.4	0.2	0.4	0.1	Low	Choose
sweet, green, raw, 1 cup	30	4.4	1.3	2.5	0.3	Low	Choose
sweet, green or red, boiled, 1 cup	38	7.4	1.2	1.6	0.3	Low	Choose
sweet, red, raw, 1 cup	39	6	1.5	3	0.5	Low	Choose
sweet, yellow, raw, 1 large pepper	50	10.1	1.9	1.7	0.4	Low	Choose
pickle, dill, 1 large	24	4	0.8	1.6	0.3	ND	Choose
pickle, sour, 1 large	15	1.5	0.5	1.6	0.3	ND	Choose
pickle, sweet, 1 large	41	10.7	0.1	0.4	0.1	ND	Choose
potato							
au gratin, 1/2 cup (100 grams)	132	9.5	5.1	1.8	7.6	ND	Restrict
boiled, w/o skin, 1 potato	118	25	2.5	2.4	0.1	Med.	Avoid
mashed, w/whole milk, butter, 1/2 cup (100 grams)	113	15.3	1.9	1.5	4.2	Med.	Restrict
potato pancake, 1 pancake	207	20.3	4.7	1.5	11.6	ND	Avoid

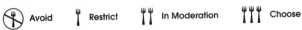

Avoid   Restrict   In Moderation   Choose

Food	Cal	Net Carb	Protein	Fiber	Total Fat	Glycemic Load	Advice
red, baked, 1 large	266	53.2	6.9	5.4	0.5	High+	🚫
russet, baked, 1 large	290	57.2	7.9	6.9	0.4	High+	🚫
white, baked, 1 large	281	56.7	6.3	6.3	0.5	High+	🚫
pumpkin, cooked, 1 cup	49	9.3	1.8	2.7	0.2	Low	♈♈♈
radishes, raw, 1 cup, sliced	19	2	0.8	1.9	0.1	ND	♈♈♈
sauerkraut, canned, 1 cup	31	2.7	1.3	3.5	0.1	ND	♈♈♈
seaweed							
agar, dried (100 grams)	306	73.2	6.2	7.7	0.3	ND	🚫
agar, raw, 2 tbsp	3	0.6	0.1	0.1	0	ND	♈♈♈
kelp, raw, 2 tbsp	4	0.9	0.2	0.1	0.1	ND	♈♈♈
spirulina, dried, 1 cup	44	3.1	8.6	0.5	1.2	ND	♈♈♈
wakame, raw, 2 tbsp	4	0.8	0.3	0.1	0.1	ND	♈♈♈
shallots, raw, 1 tbsp	7	1.7	0.3	ND	0	ND	♈♈♈
spinach, cooked, 1 cup	41	2.5	5.4	4.3	0.5	ND	♈♈♈
spinach, raw, 1 cup	7	0.4	0.9	0.7	0.1	ND	♈♈♈
squash							
acorn, cooked, 1 cup, cubed	115	20.9	2.3	9	0.3	Low	♈
butternut, cooked, 1 cup, cubed	82	21.5	1.8	ND	0.2	Low	♈
spaghetti, cooked, 1 cup	42	7.8	1	2.2	0.4	Low	♈♈♈

Food	Cal	Net Carb	Protein	Fiber	Total Fat	Glycemic Load	Advice
summer, cooked, 1 cup, sliced	36	5.3	1.6	2.5	0.6	Low	Choose
zucchini, cooked, 1 cup, sliced	29	4.6	1.2	2.5	0.1	Low	Choose
sweet potato, baked, 1 large	162	31.4	3.6	5.9	0.3	Med.	Avoid
swiss chard, cooked, 1 cup, chopped	35	3.5	3.3	3.7	0.1	ND	Choose
taro leaves, cooked, 1 cup	35	2.9	3.9	2.9	0.6	ND	Choose
taro, cooked, 1 cup, sliced	187	39	0.7	6.7	0.2	High	Avoid
tomatillo, raw, 1/2 cup, chopped	21	2.6	0.6	1.3	0.7	ND	Choose
tomato							
crushed (100 grams)	32	5.4	1.6	1.9	0.3	ND	Choose
green, raw, 1 large	42	7.3	2.2	2	0.4	ND	Choose
orange, raw, 1 tomato	18	2.5	1.3	1	0.2	ND	Choose
red, cherry, raw, 1 cup	27	4	1.3	1.8	0.3	ND	Choose
red, cooked, 1 cup	43	7.9	2.3	1.7	0.3	ND	Choose
red, raw, 1 large	33	4.9	1.6	2.2	0.4	ND	Choose
sundried, 1/2 cup	70	11.8	3.8	3.3	0.8	ND	Choose
tomato juice, canned, 6 fl oz	31	7	1.4	0.7	0.1	Low	In Moderation
tomato paste, 1 cup	215	37.7	11.3	11.8	1.2	ND	Avoid
tomato sauce, 1 cup	90	14.4	3.2	3.7	0.5	ND	Restrict

Avoid   Restrict   In Moderation   Choose

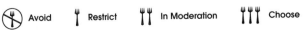

Food	Cal	Net Carb	Protein	Fiber	Total Fat	Glycemic Load	Advice
yellow, raw, 1 tomato	32	4.8	2.1	1.5	0.6	ND	♉♉♉
turnip greens, cooked, 1 cup	48	2.6	5.5	5.6	0.7	ND	♉♉♉
turnips, cooked, 1 cup, cubed	34	4.8	1.1	3.1	0.1	ND	♉♉♉
waterchestnuts, canned, 4 waterchestnuts	14	2.7	0.3	0.7	0	ND	♉♉♉
watercress, raw, 1 cup, chopped	4	0.2	0.8	0.2	0	ND	♉♉♉
yam, cooked, 1 cup, cubed	158	32.2	2	5.3	0.2	37	⊘
yellow snap beans, canned, 1/2 cup	14	2.2	0.8	0.9	0.1	ND	♉♉♉

Glossary

calorie   A measure of the amount of heat needed to raise water temperature one degree centigrade. In food, a measure of energy.

carbohydrate   One of three macronutrients in food, the others being protein and fat. Carbohydrates raise blood sugar more than any other class of food, but some carbs have a greater effect than others. Carbohydrates include simple sugars, starch, and indigestible starch (i.e., fiber) and are found in vegetables, fruits, desserts, baked goods, cereals, pastas, and all grains.

controlled-carbohydrate diet   An eating plan that limits the amount of carbohydrates in the diet, reducing the contribution of junk food and sugars.

erythritol   One of the best of the sugar alcohols, it contains 0.2 calories, a glycemic index of zero, and has no effect on blood sugar or insulin.

essential fats   Two types of fatty acids—alpha-linolenic acid and linoleic acid—that aren't made inside the body and must be obtained from the diet.

fat   One of three macronutrients in food, the others being protein and carbohydrates. Found in oils, meats, dairy, eggs, poultry, and fish, fats are categorized by their saturation. (See also *saturated fat, omega-3 fats, omega-6 fats, omega-9 fats*)

fiber   A general term for a type of carbohydrate that, for the most part, is indigestible; formerly called "roughage." Found in all plant foods. High fiber intake may reduce the risk of heart disease, diabetes, and colon cancer. (See also *insoluble fiber, soluble fiber*)

glycemic index   A measure of how fast and how high blood sugar is raised after consuming a 50-gram portion of a carbohydrate food. The scale is based on 100 for pure sucrose or white bread.

glycemic load   A measure of how fast and how high blood sugar is raised after eating a carbohydrate food, based on a specific portion size. Compared with the glycemic index, the glycemic load is a much more accurate indication of how a food will affect your blood sugar.

glycerin   A vegetable sweetener used by low-carb manufacturers to sweeten products. It has no impact on blood sugar or insulin.

insoluble fiber   Fiber that is insoluble in water. Found in wheat bran, vegetables, fruit skins, and flaxseed. Helps to quickly remove toxic waste in the colon.

insulin   A hormone secreted by the pancreas when blood sugar increases. Also known as "the hunger hormone" and "the storage hormone," insulin transports sugar from the bloodstream into cells.

inulin   A fiber used by low-carb manufacturers as a sweetener. It has no impact on blood sugar or insulin.

maltitol   A sugar alcohol with a relatively high (for sugar alcohols) glycemic index of 35. It raises blood sugar, particularly in diabetics, and can cause hunger in nondiabetics one hour after eating.

metabolic syndrome   A collection of symptoms that increase the risk of heart disease. The symptoms include: high triglycerides, low HDL cholesterol, abdominal obesity, poor blood sugar readings, and high blood pressure. Insulin resistance goes along with the syndrome, which is also sometimes called pre-diabetes.

Net Atkins Count   The phrase used by Atkins Nutritionals instead of the standard "net carbs" terminology; it claims to be more accurate than the general net carbs number.

net carbs   The total number of carbs that affect your blood sugar and insulin. The net carbs are calculated by subtracting "non-impact" carbs (i.e., fiber and sugar alcohols) from the total carbohydrate count of a food.

omega-3 fats   One of several types of unsaturated fat. There are three main omega-3 fatty acids: ALA (alpha-linolenic acid), found in flaxseed and flaxseed oil; and EPA (eicosapentaenoic acid) and DHA (docosahexaenoic acid), both found in fish. All are very healthy and important to consume.

omega-6 fats   One of several types of unsaturated fat. Omega-6s are pro-inflammatory and way too prevalent in the current standard diet.

omega-9 fats   One of several types of unsaturated fat, the very heart-healthy omega-9s are monounsaturated fats found in olive oil, nuts, and macadamia nut oils.

polydextrose   A fiber used by low-carb manufacturers as a sweetener. It has no impact on blood sugar or insulin.

protein   One of three macronutrients in food, the others being fat and carbohydrates. Composed of amino acids, proteins are essential for building structures like bones and muscles, as well as functional compounds like enzymes and neurotransmitters.

saturated fat   One of several classes of fats, saturated fat is solid at room temperature and is found in meats, poultry, dairy products, oils, and eggs.

soluble fiber   Fiber that forms a gel when mixed with liquid. Lowers cholesterol and regulates blood sugar. Found in fruits, vegetables, flaxseed, and oat bran.

sorbitol   A sugar alcohol mostly used in chewing gum and mints. Sorbitol is actually a mild cellular toxin.

sugar alcohols   A class of naturally occurring compounds similar in chemical structure to sugars. Some do not affect blood sugar and insulin at all, while others do.

trans-fats   The worst and most dangerous kind of fat, which can be identified by the phrase "partially hydrogenated oil" on a food's nutrition label.

xylitol   A sugar alcohol used in gum and as a granulated sweetener, xylitol has significant health benefits because it is antibacterial. It has a small impact on blood sugar.